W0113624

'This book extends scholarship in this area beyond the "simple and unreflexive" binary view of gender, presenting an array of contributions by leading voices in the field on issues pertinent to trans people's sexual and reproductive health.'

Dr Tracy Morison, *Massey University, New Zealand*

'We are reminded that even in light of the myriad of barriers to reproductive and sexual health and justice, trans people can and do experience joy, pleasure, happiness and euphoria.'

Dr A.J. Lowik, *Gender Equity Advisor, Centre for Gender and Sexual Health Equity, US*

'The authors reveal new pathways to justice, and indeed liberation, through an explicit focus on the experiences of trans and gender diverse people in the arena of reproductive and sexual health and rights.'

Dr. Avery Everhart, *Incoming Postdoctoral Research Fellow, School of Information and School of Public Health, University of Michigan, US*

TRANS REPRODUCTIVE AND SEXUAL HEALTH

Focusing on reproductive and sexual justice, this important book explores in detail both the challenges that trans people face when negotiating reproductive and sexual health in restrictive social contexts, and their agency in advocating for change.

Chapters cover a breadth of topics such as intimacy, sexual violence, reproductive intentions, sexuality education, oncology, and pregnancy, introducing readers to the latest research in the field as well as key emerging concepts. The authors identify core principles for trans reproductive and sexual justice, providing a broad overview of what is currently succeeding and what can be built on going into the future.

Trans Reproductive and Sexual Health offers a comprehensive exploration that is essential reading for academics and students in psychology, sociology, gender studies, and related areas, as well as clinicians and policy makers, offering direct implications for professional audiences working in health and social care.

Damien W. Riggs is a Professor in Psychology at Flinders University and an Australian Research Council Future Fellow. He is the author of over 200 publications on gender, family, and mental health.

Jane M. Ussher is Professor of Women's Health Psychology, at Western Sydney University. She has published 13 books and over 300 publications in women's sexual and reproductive health, including the health of trans people.

Kerry H. Robinson is a Professor in Sociology at Western Sydney University, Australia. Kerry has expertise in childhood, gender, and sexuality; sexuality education; and gender and sexuality-based violence and harassment and has written widely in these areas.

Shoshana Rosenberg is a butch dyke living and working on unceded Wurundjeri/Boon Wurrung land in Naarm/Melbourne. Their writing focuses on the intersections of transness, sexuality, health, sonics, and faith.

WOMEN AND PSYCHOLOGY
Series Editor: Jane M. Ussher
Professor of Women's Health Psychology, Western Sydney University

This series brings together current theory and research on women and psychology. Drawing on scholarship from a number of different areas of psychology, it bridges the gap between abstract research and the reality of women's lives by integrating theory and practice, research and policy.

Each book addresses a 'cutting edge' issue of research, covering topics such as postnatal depression and eating disorders, and addressing a wide range of theories and methodologies.

The series provides accessible and concise accounts of key issues in the study of women and psychology, and clearly demonstrates the centrality of psychology debates within women's studies or feminism.

Other titles in this series:

MOTHERING BABIES IN DOMESTIC VIOLENCE
Fiona Buchanan

BODIES THAT BIRTH
Rachelle Chadwick

JUST SEX?
Second edition
Nicola Gavey

DOMESTIC VIOLENCE AND PSYCHOLOGY
Paula Nicolson

WOMEN, SEX, AND MADNESS
Breanne Fahs

THE MATERNAL EXPERIENCE
Margo Lowy

POSTFEMINISM AND BODY IMAGE
Sarah Riley, Adrienne Evans and Martine Robson

TRANS REPRODUCTIVE AND SEXUAL HEALTH

Justice, Embodiment and Agency

Edited by Damien W. Riggs, Jane M. Ussher,
Kerry H. Robinson and Shoshana Rosenberg

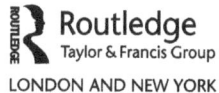

Routledge
Taylor & Francis Group

LONDON AND NEW YORK

Designed cover image: artwork by Danielle Navarro (art.djnavarro.net)

First published 2023
by Routledge
4 Park Square, Milton Park, Abingdon, Oxon OX14 4RN

and by Routledge
605 Third Avenue, New York, NY 10158

Routledge is an imprint of the Taylor & Francis Group, an informa business

© 2023 selection and editorial matter, Damien W. Riggs, Jane M. Ussher, Kerry H. Robinson and Shoshana Rosenberg; individual chapters, the contributors

The right of Damien W. Riggs, Jane M. Ussher, Kerry H. Robinson and Shoshana Rosenberg to be identified as the authors of the editorial material, and of the authors for their individual chapters, has been asserted in accordance with sections 77 and 78 of the Copyright, Designs and Patents Act 1988.

All rights reserved. No part of this book may be reprinted or reproduced or utilised in any form or by any electronic, mechanical, or other means, now known or hereafter invented, including photocopying and recording, or in any information storage or retrieval system, without permission in writing from the publishers.

Trademark notice: Product or corporate names may be trademarks or registered trademarks, and are used only for identification and explanation without intent to infringe

British Library Cataloguing-in-Publication Data
A catalogue record for this book is available from the British Library

ISBN: 978-0-367-68619-2 (hbk)
ISBN: 978-0-367-68618-5 (pbk)
ISBN: 978-1-003-13831-0 (ebk)

DOI: 10.4324/9781003138310

Typeset in Bembo
by SPi Technologies India Pvt Ltd (Straive)

CONTENTS

CONTRIBUTORS

Kimberley Allison is an Associate Research Fellow in the Translational Research Institute at Western Sydney University. She is co-author of a series of publications on LGBTQI cancer survivorship and care, as a member of the Out with Cancer Study team.

Antoinette Anazodo is a Paediatric and Adolescent Oncologist based at the Kids Cancer Centre, Sydney Children's Hospital and School of Women's and Children's, University of New South Wales, Sydney, Australia. She is co-author of a series of publications on LGBTQI cancer survivorship and care, as a member of the Out with Cancer Study team.

Clare Bartholomaeus is a Research Fellow in the Melbourne Graduate School of Education, University of Melbourne and an adjunct Research Fellow in the College of Education, Psychology and Social Work at Flinders University, South Australia. She is co-author of the book *Transgender People and Education* (with Damien W. Riggs, Palgrave Macmillan, 2017).

Eloise Brook is a writer, advocate, and academic. As an academic she has written on the formation of queer families on television. Her current research projects include trans people in public health and developing models for media representation of trans in the Media. Ella also works at the Gender Centre, Sydney.

Bella Bushby works in the HIV and public health sector and led the Trans and Gender Diverse Health and Social Needs Assessment study (the Positive Life Study). She currently works as a Senior Project Officer at the Kirby Institute, UNSW Sydney.

Rosie Charter is a Researcher and recently completed PhD scholar in the Translational Research Institute at Western Sydney University. She conducted her PhD research on trans parenting.

Teddy Cook specialises in community development, health promotion and program delivery at ACON, and is architect of TransHub. He is the Vice President of the Australian Professional Association for Trans Health and is Adjunct Lecturer at the Kirby Institute, UNSW. Teddy joins ACON's senior leadership team as a proud man of trans experience.

Jane Costello is the CEO of Positive Life NSW, a peer-led and run representative body of all people living with HIV in NSW. As a woman living with HIV, Jane is passionate about education and raising awareness around the lived experience of HIV as a way to help eliminate stigma and discrimination.

Cristyn Davies is a Research Fellow in the Specialty of Child and Adolescent Health, Faculty of Medicine and Health, University of Sydney. She has expertise in gender and sexuality; child and adolescent health and development; sexual and reproductive health; health education and comprehensive sexuality education; and knowledge translation and implementation science.

Colin Ellis is a Researcher and PhD scholar in the Translational Research Institute at Western Sydney University. He conducted his PhD research on LGBTQI cancer survivorship and care, focusing on gender and sexuality diverse men.

Alexandra J. Hawkey is a Research Fellow in the Translational Research Institute at Western Sydney University, with expertise in culturally and linguistically diverse populations. She is the co-author of a series of publications on trans sexual and reproductive health, as part of the Crossing the Line and Out with Cancer Study teams.

Martha Hickey is a Gynaecologist in the Department of Obstetrics and Gynaecology, University of Melbourne and the Royal Women's Hospital, Melbourne, Australia. She is co-author of a series of publications on LGBTQI cancer survivorship and care, as a member of the Out with Cancer Study team.

Sally Hines is a Professor in the Department of Sociological Studies at the University of Sheffield. She is the author of *Transforming gender: Transgender practices of identity, intimacy and care* (Routledge, 2007) and *Is gender fluid? A primer for the 21st century* (Thames & Hudson, 2018).

Ruth Pearce is a Lecturer in Community Development at the University of Glasgow. She is the author of *Understanding trans health: Discourse, power and* *possibilities* (Policy Press, 2018), and the co-editor of the collection *TERF Wars: Feminism and the fight for transgender futures* (Sage, 2020).

Janette Perz is Professor and Director of the Translational Research Institute at Western Sydney University. She has 25 years experience in research on sexual and reproductive health and is the co-author of a series of publications on LGBTQI cancer survivorship and trans sexual violence.

Chloe Parton is a Lecturer in the School of Health, Te Herenga Waka – Victoria University of Wellington. She has expertise in women's embodiment, and is the co-author of a series of publications on LGBTQI cancer survivorship and care, as a member of the Out with Cancer Study team.

Carla A. Pfeffer is a Professor in the School of Social Work at Michigan State University. She is the author of *Queering families: The postmodern partnerships of cisgender women and transgender men* (Oxford University Press, 2016).

Rosalie Power is an Associate Research Fellow in the Translational Research Institute at Western Sydney University. She is co-author of a series of publications on LGBTQI cancer survivorship and care, as a member of the Out with Cancer Study team.

Damien W. Riggs is a Professor in Psychology at Flinders University and an Australian Research Council Future Fellow. He is the author of over 200 publications on gender, family, and mental health, including (with Shoshana Rosenberg, Heather Fraser, and Nik Taylor) *Queer entanglements: Gender, sexuality and animal companionship* (Cambridge University Press, 2021).

Kerry H. Robinson is a Professor in Sociology in the School of Social Sciences, at Western Sydney University. Kerry is currently researching gender, gender equity policy and practice in schools; sexual harassment of LGBTQ young people in the workplace; and being trans in the early years. Kerry is a member of the Out with Cancer study team.

Shoshana Rosenberg is an Independent Researcher currently based in Naarm/ Melbourne, Victoria. Their research has focused on trans peoples' experiences of pleasure, embodiment, and sexual health. Shoshana is an Associate Editor at the *International Journal of Transgender Health*, and has recently published a co-authored manuscript (*Queer Entanglements*) through Cambridge University Press.

Chantell Sheehan is currently a Clinical Psychology Registrar. She splits her time by working in private practice that centres on trauma and eating related presentations, and an NGO focusing on youth mental health. She conducted analysis of the Positive Life Study data as part of her Master's in Clinical Psychology research, based at Western Sydney University.

Rachel Skinner is a Professor in Paediatrics, in the Faculty of Medicine and Health, Sydney University, and Deputy Director of *Wellbeing, Health and Youth* (why.org. au), a National Health and Medical Research Council funded Centre of Research Excellence in Adolescent Health. She is a paediatrician and specialist in Adolescent and Young Adult Medicine at the Children's Hospital Westmead in Sydney.

Samantha Sperring is a Researcher and PhD scholar in the Translational Research Institute at Western Sydney University. She conducted her PhD research on LGBTQI cancer survivorship and care, focusing on gender and sexuality diverse women.

Jane M. Ussher is Professor of Women's Health Psychology, at Western Sydney University. She has published 13 books and over 300 publications in women's sexual and reproductive health, including the health of trans people. She is co-author of a series of publications on trans sexual and reproductive health, as lead investigator on the Crossing the Line and Out with Cancer Study teams.

Francis Ray White is a Senior Lecturer in Social Science at the University of Westminster. Their research, writing and teaching is in the area of gender studies, particularly around questions of queer, trans, and fat embodiment.

ACKNOWLEDGEMENTS

The authors acknowledge that they live on the unceded lands of the Kaurna people, the Gadigal people, the Dharawal people, and the people of the Kulin Nations. We acknowledge their sovereignty as First Nations people.

Thanks to Danielle Navarro for providing the cover art for this book. Danielle's work is available at https://art.djnavarro.net.

1

INTRODUCTION

Damien W. Riggs, Jane M. Ussher, Kerry H. Robinson and Shoshana Rosenberg

Defining reproductive and sexual health

Reproductive health deals with reproductive processes, functions, and systems at all stages of life, and is a crucial part of general health and human development (World Health Organization, 2014). As the World Health Organization (WHO) states, "reproductive health is a state of complete physical, mental and social well-being and not merely the absence of disease or infirmity". Implicit in this are the rights of individuals to be informed and to have access to safe, effective, affordable, and acceptable regulation of fertility, the right of access to appropriate health care services that will enable individuals to go safely through pregnancy and childbirth with the best chance of having a healthy infant, and absence of reproductive coercion (Ussher, Chrisler, & Perz, 2020).

A complex array of factors is implicated in reproductive health, conceptualised in the context of a person's age, gender, and socioeconomic, cultural, and political environments. Principal among these is the place of an individual in society, particularly in terms of their control over their own bodies, reproductive choices, and access to education. But other issues also contribute to how individuals experience reproductive health. This includes systemic and/or structural issues, such as health service provision, privacy and confidentiality, and representations in the media of normative reproductive bodies (Hankivsky, Cormier, & De Merich, 2009; Ussher, 2006). It also includes risk factors, such as violence, abuse of drugs or alcohol, and powerlessness to control reproductive health (McKenzie-Mohr & Lafrance, 2014). Finally, reproductive health is influenced by psychosocial factors, such as beliefs and expectations associated with reproduction, individuals' experiences of their bodies, and their self-confidence and self-esteem (Tolman, Bowman, & Fahs, 2014).

Sexual health is closely related to reproductive health. Yet while sexual health and reproductive health are closely related, sexual health advocacy often treats

DOI: 10.4324/9781003138310-1

sexual health as a distinct matter, so as to ensure that sexual health is not reduced to matters of disease, and instead also encompasses pleasure and sexual wellbeing (Gruskin et al., 2019). This is reflected in the WHO (1994) definition of sexual health, which explicitly refers to "the enhancement of life and personal relations, and not merely counselling and care related to reproduction and sexually transmitted diseases". A focus on sexual pleasure is vital to work in the field of sexual health. Similar to work in the field of reproductive health, which focuses not simply on health and access, but also on the right to make decisions about reproduction and for individuals to determine what reproduction might or might not look like for them (such as including the right to abortion), a focus on sexual pleasure ensures that sexual health encompasses the right to make decisions about sexual intimacy, and the capacity to enact such decisions.

This focus on agentic decision making as part of reproductive and sexual health is vital, so as to counter what Tuck (2009) refers to as 'damage centered research'. Tuck defines damage-centred research as research that focuses only on deficit, requiring marginalised communities specifically to frame their experiences in terms of harms caused by marginalisation. As Tuck notes, it is certainly important to focus on the harm caused by marginalisation: both in its historical forms (i.e., colonisation, slavery), and in the implications of historical forms upon contemporary experiences. Yet as Tuck further notes, the contextualisation of marginalisation as part of the experience of marginalised communities all too often results in harm caused being treated as the most salient feature of any marginalised community. Such a focus on harm not only fails to focus on strengths, resistance, and indeed joy, but it also treats harm as inherent to marginalised communities, in effect constituting damage-centred research as pathologising research.

Further, with regard to damage-centred research on reproductive and sexual health specifically, Tuck (2009) suggests that in order to warrant their inclusion, marginalised communities are often expected to repeatedly share stories about harms caused, in order to justify to those in power that change should occur (i.e., increased rights). Such an approach to social change is problematic for multiple reasons. First, it brings with it the capacity to re-traumatise people for whom trauma is their experience of marginalisation. Second, it infers that the public record is not already replete with evidence of harms caused, instead suggesting that yet more evidence is required. Third, it requires marginalised people to in effect litigate their own marginalisation via narratives of harm. This places responsibility upon individual people, rather than upon the state to provide redress.

Both Mama (2002) and Brown (2020) have similarly noted that the injunction to evidence harm becomes a founding narrative for marginalised communities. One consequence of this is that members of marginalised communities who are unwilling to provide narratives of harm, or who refuse to litigate their own experiences of marginalisation (instead expecting the state to provide redress), are treated as inauthentic marginalised group members. In terms of sexual health, for example, people who experience sexual violence and who do not experience this as traumatising are treated as inauthentic victims (Gavey & Schmidt, 2011). In terms of reproductive health, for example, cisgender women who request hysterectomies at a young age are treated as not capable of knowing their own reproductive desires (in contrast to young cisgender women with disabilities, incarcerated cisgender women, and cisgender women of a diversity of cultural and socioeconomic groups, who continue to be subjected to hysterectomies against their will). In both of these examples, standardised narratives of reproductive and sexual health create damage-centred norms to which all people are expected to adhere, and a refusal to adhere may be treated as a refusal of membership of a particular social class. As we explore later in this chapter, challenging damage-centred research is thus vital, part of which requires situating harms experienced alongside strengths and accounts of agency.

Reproductive and sexual health research has historically focused on the bodies of cisgender women and men, distinguished from each other across a simple and unreflexive binary. 'Woman' has been taken to mean a female with a cervix and ovaries; 'man', a male with a penis and testes. Trans people, and those with intersex variations, are almost invisible within this narrow dichotomy. This means that whole groups of people are excluded from reproductive and sexual health research and health care, such as cervical cancer screening (Connolly, Hughes, & Berner, 2020), in vitro fertilisation (Riggs & Bartholomaeus, 2019), pregnancy support (Charter, Ussher, Perz, & Robinson, 2018), and contraception (Light, Wang, Zeymo, & Gomez-Lobo, 2018). In recent years there has been a growing recognition of the complexity of gender in relation to reproductive and sexual health, and need to address the reproductive and sexual health of trans people. For example, in critical menstruation studies, the use of the term 'menstruators' rather than 'women who have periods' acknowledges that many trans people bleed once a month (Rydström, 2020). Inclusive language is also recommended in relation to menopause (Gender GP, 2021a), cervical screening (Gender GP, 2021b), and pregnancy (Obedin-Maliver & Makadon, 2016), amongst other areas. Consideration of the reproductive and sexual health of trans people needs to move from the margins, to be part of the central core of theory, research, and practice.

The importance of addressing reproductive and sexual health across the lifespan

It is important that a lifespan approach is taken to reproductive and sexual health that includes addressing the needs and early education of young people and children. There is limited research that includes young people's perspectives about fertility, fertility preservation, sexual health, and other aspects of their future reproductive lives. This is particularly so for trans young people. Socio-cultural discourses of childhood and sexuality underpin some adults' views that addressing reproductive and sexual health information with young people, especially children, is 'developmentally age inappropriate' and thus, irrelevant to their lives. These perceptions are generally reflected in the controversial nature of children's and young people's access to inclusive sexuality education (Robinson, 2013; Robinson, Smith & Davies, 2017). Discourses of childhood also impact perceptions of children's and young people's ability to make decisions about their lives – including about their bodies. However, reproductive, and sexual health information is relevant to children and young people and to their health and wellbeing, particularly to trans children and young people. Trans young people are required to make important decisions early in life about their reproductive futures when making decisions about gender affirming hormones. Trans and sexuality diverse young people are also more likely than cisgender young people to be sexually active earlier, contract sexually transmitted infections, and become pregnant (Hillier et al., 2010). Trans young people are generally not accessing sexuality education, inclusive of reproductive and sexual health issues pertinent to their needs (Riggs & Bartholomaeus, 2018; Shannon, 2022).

Defining reproductive and sexual justice

As noted in the first section of this chapter, fundamental to reproductive and sexual health is the language of rights: ensuring that legislation enshrines the right to self-determination, and that public policy and services make possible avenues to enact rights. By contrast, a focus on reproductive and sexual *justice* emphasises the potential gap between rights and the possibility of enacting rights (Ross & Solinger, 2017). In other words, it is one thing for legislation to exist that gives rights to groups of people with regard to their reproductive and sexual health. It is another thing entirely for policies and services to exist that enable people to enact the rights that they hold. Consider an example. A person may live in a state or country that legislates for abortion rights. But if the state or country does not provide abortion services, or only provides user-pays services (as opposed to public health care), or utilises terminology in policy that limits abortions to particular people or a particular gestational age, then the capacity of individuals to enact the rights they hold is seriously curtailed. The concept of reproductive justice (as first developed by a collective of Black women named 'Women of African Descent for Reproductive Justice' in 1994) and by extension the concept of sexual justice thus calls for attention to the ways in which rights are constrained by institutions and ideologies.

Reproductive and sexual justice thus focuses on how societies may not be inclusive, even if laws may be. Consider the example where a single heterosexual woman may have the right to access assisted reproductive technologies, but where she is shamed for being a single mother by her community. Reproductive and sexual justice also focuses on how *services* may not be inclusive, even if laws may be. Consider the example where a gay couple may have the right to marriage, but when they approach a pastry chef to make their wedding cake, the chef declines to provide services to a gay couple on the basis of a religious objection. Reproductive and sexual justice, then, speaks to social norms, and how they serve to limit the enactment of reproductive and sexual rights. To give another example, reproductive and sexual health, framed through the lens of rights, might emphasise the rights of people to have children if they wish to. But the enactment of such rights is premised upon living conditions that impact upon whether or not someone's reproductive health is compromised. It is premised upon histories of marginalisation that shape an individual's parenting capacity. It is premised upon how particular marginalised individuals are at increased risk of having their children removed under child protection laws. And it is premised upon the capacity to raise children who live healthy lives, who themselves are not subject to unnecessary state intervention, and indeed whose lives are cut short by inadequate social care. The right to have children is thus a basic right. But sitting alongside that are a spectrum of practices as well as rights that determine whether or not the having of a child will result in being able to raise that child, and indeed whether or not the child (and their parents) live to enjoy a happy life (Ross & Solinger, 2017).

While the example above with regard to having children to a certain degree emphasises reproductive justice, sexual justice is equally important. Sexual justice, using again the example of having a child, pertains not simply to the right to consent to reproduction, and specifically sex, but also the capacity to reproduce at a time of one's choosing, to do so with a partner (if that is desired) who is supportive and caring, to not have one's fertility used as a form of control (both by a partner and by the state), to enact one's sexuality in a positive way as a parent, and to teach one's children about sexual rights, sexual health, and sexual justice (Gruskin et al., 2019). While in a given state or country an individual may have the right to sexual self-determination (and this is not the case in all states or countries, such as where rape in the context of marriage is not a crime in all states or countries), they may not have access to affordable contraception that enables them to choose when or if to reproduce. Social policies and services may fail to provide information to support people to negotiate intimacy after the arrival of a child. So too they may fail to provide information for parents to teach their children about sexual safety, or may do so solely from an abstinence-based model. These factors thus limit an individual's capacity to enact their sexual rights.

Richardson (2000) outlines multiple forms of sexual rights that may or may not be met in any given state or country, and which require a sexual justice approach. As Richardson notes, sexual practices may be regulated according to the gender or number of partners, the types of intimacy engaged in, the location where intimacy is engaged in, and whether intimacy is paid for. While sexual rights may allow for the right to self-determination about one's own pleasure, these may be limited, for example, if one lives in a location where one's attractions are outlawed (for example if there is no legislative protection for people who are not heterosexual in terms of hate speech). Again, then, a sexual justice approach emphasises institutional constraints that may limit the extent to which an individual can enact their rights to pleasure and intimacy.

A useful way to think about reproductive and sexual justice is in terms of citizenship. Here citizenship is not limited to whether or not someone is a legal citizen of a particular state or country, though it does encompass that. Rather, citizenship refers to an individual's capacity to engage in activities in ways that accord with those typically expected for other people living in the same state or country. Further, citizenship pertains to what is normatively expected of individuals living in a specific state or country: what is expected of people in terms of how they act, what they believe, and in the context of this book, the sexual and reproductive lives that they seek to live. The terms 'sexual' or 'intimate' citizenship have been developed to account for the lives that people are expected to live in terms of sexuality (Richardson, 2017), and the term 'reproductive citizenship' has developed to account for the lives that people are expected to live in terms of reproduction (Turner, 2001).

Work in the area of sexual or intimate citizenship has often focused closely on the right to privacy, thus positioning sexuality as a private matter (Richardson, 2017). While this has been effective in some contexts in terms of removing state control from the private lives of individuals, it has also served to reinforce the idea that the regulation of intimacy is a private matter, not of concern to the state. For people subject to sexual coercion, for example, and particularly in the context of intimate relationships, the framing of sexuality as a private matter can make allegations of coercion in intimate relationships particularly hard to adjudicate. In many ways the rendering of sexuality as a private matter is in direct contradiction to the idea of citizenship, and specifically in terms of an individual's place within the body politic. This contradiction, however, is made intelligible by the framing of the *regulation* of sexuality as a public matter, and the *enactment* of sexuality as a private matter. This distinction, however, often fails to provide sufficient protection over matters considered private, as much as it treats as public matters that are deemed not protected by the right to privacy. The example above with regard to sexual coercion in intimate relationships provides an example of the former. With regard to the latter, in many states or countries it was only relatively recently that non-heterosexual intimacy was considered a private matter, and even in those locations where non-heterosexual intimacy is now protected by law, public discourse about such intimacy is still often reliant upon narratives of indecency.

In terms of reproductive justice and citizenship, the distinction between public and private is perhaps even more acute. This is especially true with regard to the regulation of women's bodies. On the one hand, the example above of sexual coercion is often especially felt by women. Statistics on (primarily cisgender) women's experiences of domestic violence, for example, highlight that relegating intimate relationships to the private sphere can mean that such women are left without adequate protection. On the other hand, the public regulation of cisgender women's reproductive and sexual bodies suggests that such women in particular are seen as subjected to heightened public scrutiny. Consider debates over cisgender women breastfeeding in public, or discussions about cisgender women's clothing being included in deliberations about rape in public places. These examples highlight the fact that, as much as women, for example, may be failed by the state in terms of protections in the private sphere, they are equally overregulated in the public sphere on the basis of public opinion and normative assumptions. Ignored in all of these conversations, and as we will explore below, are trans people's experiences of each of the phenomena outlined above. If cisgender women's experiences of domestic violence are framed in particular marginalising ways, then this is exacerbated for many trans people. Similarly, if breastfeeding is fraught for many cisgender women, consider the experiences of trans masculine people chestfeeding in public.

Beasley and Bacchi (2000) suggest that part of the problem of the public/private divide is a product of the focus on citizenship as a primarily public affair, comprised of purportedly agreed upon public standards, conventions, and beliefs. Indeed, these three forms of purportedly agreed upon aspects of citizenship highlight that the equation of citizenship with public life is reliant upon the idea that public life refers almost exclusively to instrumentalised, rationalised, public thought and action. Left out of this narrative of citizenship is the body: the public body and the individual body. Both intimate or sexual citizenship and reproductive citizenship as concepts attempt to bring the body back into discussions of citizenship, yet as Beasley and Bacchi argue, the body is often still conceptualised as a private matter, stripped of all aspects of what they refer to as 'social flesh'.

For Beasley and Bacchi (2007), 'social flesh' evokes a political metaphor that emphasises new ways of thinking about the intersections of human bodies and the body politic. It challenges the idea of the individual citizen enacting (or not) rights determined by the state, and instead emphasises the idea that both interpersonal relationships, and relationships between the individuals and the state, are fleshy experiences. Here the term flesh does not refer simply to the human body, but rather to how relationships between humans and between humans and the state are given 'thickness' or 'flesh' by a plethora of social norms, legislative practices, embodied experiences, and individual interactions. More specifically, and as it pertains to reproductive and sexual justice, 'social flesh' places emphasis on how particular bodies (both individuals and states) are positioned as either in control or out of control, and thus how bodies must either regulate or be regulated. As Beasley and Bacchi argue, the point, however, is not to simply repeat these binaries. Rather, it is to examine their imbrication. To be positioned as out of control is to be framed by a system that seeks to control. Being out of control is not inherent to a particular body, but is rather a product of citizenship claims that produce particular forms of intelligible citizenship.

Sexual citizenship is important to children and young people, as it is to adults. The idea that sexual citizenship has relevance to children and young people's lives is often met with resistance and hostility by some adults, who view it as inappropriately crossing the adult/child binary boundary. Children's and young people's sexual citizenship is about: access to information about bodies, relationships, reproduction, and sexual health; learning to become agentic ethical gendered and sexual subjects and to respect gender and sexuality diversity; having an awareness and understanding of their rights as sexual subjects; to be supported in building confidence and resilience to become informed sexual subjects; and fostering their health and well-being (Robinson, 2022). Children and young people's access to ongoing relevant and inclusive sexuality education throughout their lives is central to the building of sexual citizenship early in life. All these issues are particularly relevant to the lives of trans children and young people.

Importantly, and as Beasley and Bacchi (2007) note, the concept of social flesh is not a proxy for gender, even if often in their work it has focused specifically on cisgender women. Rather, social flesh accounts for how all institutions and individuals are mutually regulated, even if in differing ways. As the examples we have already given in this chapter would suggest, reproductive and sexual rights are differentially available to individuals, they are differentially enacted, produce differentiated claims to and about citizenship, and require differing responses from a reproductive and sexual justice framework. As we shall see in the following section, and as we introduced briefly in the first section of this chapter, to date the focus of sexual and reproductive health, and by extension sexual and reproductive justice, has largely focused on particular cohorts of cisgender women. Yet as this book stands as a testament, sexual and reproductive justice frameworks have clear import for a diversity of groups.

Trans people and reproductive and sexual justice

Thus far in this chapter we have focused broadly on reproductive and sexual justice for all people. This book, however, focuses specifically on reproductive and sexual justice for trans people. As we noted in the previous section, a focus on reproductive and sexual justice is often necessary given that in many contexts rights do not automatically translate into material or institutional gain for marginalised individuals. This is especially true with regard to trans people, given the effects of cisgenderism. Cisgenderism is defined as "the discriminatory ideology that delegitimises people's own designations of their genders and bodies" (Ansara & Hegarty, 2013, p. 162). Forms of cisgenderism include failing or refusing to use a person's name or pronouns (i.e., misgendering), presuming that assigned sex determines gender, treating gender diversity as a pathology, presuming that there are only two genders, and treating the topic of gender diversity as taboo.

As the above definition of cisgenderism would suggest, key is the idea that there is a relationship between assigned sex and gender. It is typically presumed that a person assigned female at birth will experience their gender as female, and that a person assigned male at birth will experience their gender as male. Yet this presumption is flawed in many ways as a result of cisgenderism. The referent 'assigned sex' is a historically and culturally dependent descriptor used to group individuals into one of two categories (female or male), ignoring considerable diversity between members of either group, and excluding people for whom neither group is wholly applicable. Further, while the referent 'assigned sex' is notionally attached to a constellation of bodily configurations (primarily with regard to primary and secondary sex characteristics, but also including chromosomal makeup), the referent 'gender' speaks to a psychological concept pertaining to how we understand ourselves in relation to available categories of difference, again all of which is historically and culturally contingent.

Given the contingency of the referents 'assigned sex' and 'gender', it is reasonable to suggest that both are problematic for all people, given they are reliant upon culturally determined points of difference that are treated as salient, that there is considerable diversity among supposed groups of people, and that they are ultimately exclusionary. Nonetheless, cisgenderism functions via the presumption that there is some sort of relationship between sex and gender, treating as typical those people whose experience of their gender relates in a normative way to their assigned sex. This majority group of people are referred to as cisgender. For a minority group of people, the cisgenderist logic that assigned sex determines gender is shown to be false. In this book, we refer to this group of people using the umbrella term 'trans'. This diverse group includes people with a binary gender (i.e., female or male), and people with a non-binary gender (inclusive of people whose gender is fluid, whose gender is nonbinary, or who have no experience of having a gender). Importantly, and given our critique above of the historical and cultural depending of the category 'assigned sex', we refuse the common injunction to reserve the terms 'female' and 'male' to refer to sexed bodies, instead affirming the appropriateness of, for example, referring to trans women as female. This is in addition to using experience-specific language to refer to certain phenomena, rather than tying them to specific genders or sexed bodies (such as referring to 'people who menstruate').

When applying concepts of reproductive and sexual justice to the lives of trans people, then, it is vital to focus on how cisgenderism shapes experiences of reproductive and sexual rights. As Pearce (2018) notes, trans people in the context of health care are often viewed within a binary of either having a 'condition' that needs fixing, or as constituting a movement, both in the sense of a social movement, and as 'moving' between sex and gender categories. While this binary is framed as oppositional, as Pearce notes in many ways it forms a complementary whole, one in which trans people are framed as exceptions to a cisgenderist rule. As a result, reproductive and sexual rights often either fail to speak to the needs of trans people entirely, or include trans people as an 'add on' to an existing cisgenderist logic. Again, it is for these reasons that a trans reproductive and sexual justice approach is vital.

Historically, as we will explore in more detail later in this chapter, for many trans people reproductive and sexual justice has focused primarily on the right to be alive. In the face of cisgenderist logics, including those that have sanctioned (and continue to sanction) necropolitical understandings of trans people's lives, trans people continue to fight for the right to live. Yet as cárdenas (2016) argues, reproductive and sexual justice must constitute more than just the right to live. This is not to ignore that for many trans people the fight is simply to be recognised as humans the same as cisgender people, and to be allowed to make determinations about their lives as would any person. But as this book is a testament, there are many areas of reproductive and sexual justice that require focused attention beyond simply the right to live and be seen as human.

The tension here, then, is to navigate a path through an understanding of reproductive and sexual justice for trans people that is mindful of specificities, as well as acknowledging that such specificities are produced by cisgenderism. In other words, and as we will explore in the following sections of this chapter, there are many areas of reproductive and sexual justice approaches that take specific forms when applied to the lives of trans people. Yet these specificities, we would argue, are not a product of something unique inherent to trans people absent of the broader social context in which they live. Rather, the specific needs of trans people with regard to reproductive and sexual health are a product of how cisgenderism shapes and often limits people's lives. To put it another way: trans people's lives are all too often framed as exceptional or marginal because cisgenderism frames them as such. Our argument here is not that trans people's lives cannot be exceptional and are not often framed by marginalisation; rather, and as part of a trans reproductive and sexual justice approach, what is needed are ways of seeing trans people as part of a broader humanity united by resistance to inequality in all forms.

Take as an example the case of gender affirmation in the form of health care. All too often, receiving gender affirming medical treatment is framed as constituting a 'special need' sought out by trans people. As Gruskin et al. (2018) argue, being affirmed in one's gender, and receiving medical responses (if desired) that further affirm one's gender, are hard fought for gains experienced by some (but not all) trans people. As we explore below, affirming medical treatment produces reproductive and sexual health gains for trans people. Yet such 'gains' only serve to place trans people on par with their cisgender peers: they are not 'special rights', but rather constitute rights in the form of access to affirming medical care that enable some trans people to live fulfilling lives similar to their cisgender peers. To view the receipt of affirming medical care as exceptional is to ignore the effects of cisgenderism, and indeed to suggest that trans people should not receive care that is attentive to their reproductive and sexual health needs.

Needed, then, is a sexual and reproductive justice approach that neither erases trans people's specific experiences or needs, nor fails to attend to how cisgenderism produces trans people's experiences and needs. To date, much of the literature on reproductive and sexual justice for trans people has focused primarily on fertility preservation, access to affirming medical care, the right to be safe from harm, and the right to reproduce and safely raise children. All of these areas, we would argue, while vital, are required simply in order to combat cisgenderism. Fertility preservation continues to be an important focus given that in 14 countries trans people must 'consent' to sterilisation in order to receive gender-affirming care and to change their gender marker (Transgender Europe, 2019). Access to affirming medical care, while still patchy, is vital to counter decades of pathologising medical care forced upon trans people (Bauer et al., 2009; Riggs et al., 2019). The right to be safe from sexual violence continues to be a pressing issue, given the murder and marginalisation of trans people across the globe, and specifically trans women of colour (Transgender Europe, 2020). A focus on the right to reproduce is a consequence of forced sterilisation, as is the right to safely raise children, given that trans people still face the threat of having their children removed from them (Carter, 2006).

These areas of focus have been and continue to be vital due to the effects of cisgenderism. Yet at the same time we must ask how their centrality produces a particular norm, one increasingly referred to as transnormativity (Vipond, 2015). Transnormativity refers to the assumption that all trans people want to medically transition. It refers to the assumption that all trans people want to be 'just like' cisgender people, and specifically that they will have a binary gender and present their gender in a normative fashion. It refers to the assumption that all trans people are heterosexual, want to have children, want to marry, and want to live a life relatively unmarked by gender diversity. Certainly for some trans people all of these may be true, and that is completely fine. But for other people it may not be possible or desirable. Transnormativity, as repeated through a particularly limited (even if necessary) understanding of reproductive and sexual justice, thus serves to marginalise other equally important areas of reproductive and sexual justice. Many of these marginalised areas are our focus within this book, alongside some of the more commonly explored areas outlined above.

Finally, and as we noted in the previous section, any account of trans reproductive and sexual justice must attend to citizenship. In some contexts and times, the citizenship of trans people has and continues to be fraught, such as with regard to legal gender recognition. A lack of legal recognition has clear implications for reproductive and sexual rights. Yet even with recognition, actual reproductive and sexual justice can lag behind. Consider the example of a transgender man who is legally recognised as a man, but who struggles to access reproductive and sexual health services for a pap smear, because the services available are incapable of acknowledging that men might need pap smears. Reproductive and sexual citizenship for trans people is thus as much about legal rights as it is about the right to be seen as a legitimate part of the body politic, to have one's gender reflected in the world more broadly, to receive services that are inclusive, to not be made a focus of other people's prurient or pathologising interest, and to expect one's needs to be met as par for the course, rather than as an exceptional case or special need.

To use Beasley and Bacchi's (2007) account of social flesh, then, a focus on cisgenderism allows us to explore how trans people are alternately excluded from the body politic, or included on specific pathologising terms. A 'thicker' understanding of sociality and responsibility for trans people as part of a reproductive and sexual justice approach requires a critique of cisgenderism that examines it at all levels: from the most mundane to the explicitly discriminatory and violent; from the interpersonal to the institutional. The issue at stake, then, is not how to better regulate trans people's lives, or perhaps not even how to regulate for trans people. Rather, it is to examine how the state by default excludes trans people from civic society, as a result of cisgenderism. Rather than 'add on' approaches that tinker at the edges, then, a trans reproductive and sexual justice approach must fundamentally rethink how we conceptualise justice. To that end, in the following two sections we first explore barriers to trans reproductive and sexual justice, and then explore areas of focus that facilitate trans reproductive and sexual justice.

Barriers to trans reproductive and sexual justice

A key barrier to trans sexual justice specifically pertains to the alternating desexualisation and hypersexualisation of trans people. Historically, as Latham (2019) explores, trans people presenting for medical treatment were expected not simply to present as having a binary gender and being heterosexual, but more specifically to present as having little to no sexual desire; given, historically, most medical treatment was directed toward trans women, and the requirement of presenting a desexualised sense of self was intended to ward against accusations of homosexuality, but also to move trans women outside of the body politic proper, and instead to position trans women at best as an adjunct to a normative femininity. Trans women were expected both to be model representations of a normative femininity, while at the same time reporting no sexual desire. Indeed, desire was expected to focus on gender transition, rather than any potential intimate desire that may accompany gender transition.

As trans people, and trans women in particular, increasingly came to public attention from the 1950s onwards, however, the medical requirement of desexualisation has been accompanied by both a public and private focus on trans women as hypersexualised. As Serano (2007) argues,

> trans women are hypersexualized in our culture because we are viewed as enabling our own sexual objectification (by virtue of the fact that we physically transition from male to female) in much the same way that a woman who wears a low-cut dress is presumed to facilitate her own objectification.
>
> *(p. 258)*

Serano further argues that public narratives about trans women and sexualisation actually sit closely alongside medical narratives of desexualisation: requirements of presenting a desexualised sense of self actually demonstrate a hyper focus on trans women's sexuality.

As both Serano and Lefebvre (2020) note, the sexualisation of trans women in particular is fraught. Not only does it overdetermine trans women's sexuality, resulting in a plethora of sexualised images of trans women in the media, in pornography, and in the expectations of potential intimate partners, but it also inculcates trans women into a logic of normative femininity, in which sexual desirability is a hallmark. As Lefebvre notes, for many trans women, while hyper sexualisation is undesirable, it nonetheless signals for some women that their gender transition is 'successful': that it has resulted in attracting the attention of others, and in particular men. However, for some trans women this can be experienced as a form of fetishisation (Ussher et al., 2022). Conversely, Serano suggests that some trans people, as a way of countering the sexualisation of their lives, seek to minimise or deny their own sexual desires. Again, then, the sexualisation of trans people's lives has direct implications for sexual justice, in that it either requires conformity to a normative understanding of trans sexuality and desire (i.e., to appeal to others), or it encourages some people to deny their desires and attractions.

Related to the hyper sexualisation of trans people is the enactment of violence, including sexual violence, against trans people. As we noted above, trans women of colour in particular are subjected to high levels of violence including murder.

Research on trans women of colour and experiences of sexual violence suggests cisgender men in particular often frame themselves as being 'entitled' to trans women's bodies, an entitlement wrapped up in cisgenderism, sexism, colonialism, and racism (Riggs & Toone, 2017; Ussher et al., 2020b). With regard to cisgenderism specifically, sexual violence is often framed by cisgender men as a 'compliment': as showing that trans women can be seen as desirable. Importantly, trans men and gender diverse people assigned female at birth are also at times located within a similar logic. The case of Branden Teena, for example, demonstrates that 'corrective rape' and ultimately murder continue to be used as mechanisms by which to control bodies read as female (Halberstam, 2005).

In many ways, the above accounts of desexualisation, hyper sexualisation, and sexual violence all encompass a focus on the reduction of trans people to mere bodies, stripped of humanity, desire, and rights. This reduction of trans people to a form of bare life made possible within a necropolitical logic in which some humans are deemed intelligible and valid, and other humans deemed less than human and thus invalid or not valued, is reflected in the logic of eugenics. Writers such as Lowik (2018) and Amin (2018) argue that a eugenics logic is reflected not simply in facts such as the forced sterilisation of trans people, both historically and in some contexts in the present; eugenics is evident more broadly in cisgenderist logics that frame which trans bodies are deemed acceptable (i.e., those that have medically transitioned, those who have a binary gender, those whose gender presentation is normative, and those who do not challenge cisgenderism). As we noted above, transnormativity endorses a very particular version of being trans. Transnormativity also endorses a eugenics logic, one in which outside the narrow boundaries of transnormativity, other trans lives are not valued.

More broadly, histories of gender diversity are enmeshed with histories of eugenics. As Amin (2018) has cogently demonstrated, histories of gender affirming surgeries are intertwined with histories of surgeries aimed at 'glandular rejuvenation', specifically the transplantation of the gonads of younger healthy people into older people. The older people who were recipients of such treatments were typically wealthy white men whose value was overdetermined within a particular racialised logic. That the treatments they received came at the expense of people subjected to sterilisation (i.e., through the removal and transplantation of their gonads) highlights how eugenics played a role in these early treatments. That these treatments then provided a medical basis for the treatment for trans people suggests not per se that trans people are complicit with eugenics, but rather that the operations of eugenics have shifting targets that have both benefited and served to regulate trans people. In other words, at the same time as some trans have been and continue to be subjected to state-sanctioned forms of bodily control with regard to reproductive and sexual rights, other trans people benefit from treatments founded in eugenics. Reconciling these two responses to trans people is possible by focusing on how trans people are too often reduced to their bodies, a practice that more recently has been challenged by a focus on trans people's rights to reproductive and sexual justice.

Facilitators of trans reproductive and sexual justice

As a counter to damage-centred ideologies that reduce trans people to pathologising accounts of their bodies, over the past decade research, particularly that conducted by trans people, has sought to emphasise pleasure, intimacy, and joy in the lives of trans people. In some cases the approach has been to normalise trans people's intimate lives, and indeed to advocate for the right of trans people to enjoy intimacy, while other approaches have sought to emphasise the potentially unique aspects of trans people's experiences of intimacy and pleasure.

In terms of pleasure, Lindley and colleagues (2020b) argue that much of the research on trans people has focused almost exclusively on people who have undertaken gender affirming medical treatment, and that such research has provided relatively normative accounts of gendered pleasure (such that trans women are depicted as having typically 'feminine' experiences of pleasure, and trans men as having typically 'masculine' experiences of pleasure). Ignored in this research are people who have not medically transitioned. Lindley and colleagues emphasise the fact that for this group of people, affirming responses from partners are key. Specifically, affirming responses from intimate partners allow trans people who have not medically transitioned to enjoy their bodies in ways that may counter experiences of dysphoria. Conversely, Lindley and colleagues (2020a) have also found that sexual dissatisfaction often related to fears that a potential intimate partner would not be affirming, or that they would fetishise the person's body.

Focusing on trans women who have received affirming medical treatment, Rosenberg et al. (2019) provide a critical account of this group of women, and in so doing resist the idea that trans women must or do experience normatively feminine modes of pleasure. Echoing the work of the zine *Fucking Trans Women* (Bellweather, 2010), Rosenberg and colleagues challenge the idea that all trans women in receipt of hormones specifically experience diminished sexual arousal. Instead, Rosenberg and colleagues emphasise that for some women forms of arousal shifted to new areas, while for other women existing forms of arousal are retained. As they suggest, desexualised narratives of trans women, often still evident in research and public narratives about the effects of hormones, fail to account for the diversity of women's experiences.

Closely related to the topic of pleasure is the topic of desire, constituting an important avenue of consideration in terms of sexual justice for trans people. Tompkins (2014) provides an extensive discussion about the role of desire in terms of cisgender partners of trans people. Challenging the idea that all such partners are by default seeking to fetishise trans people, Tompkins argues that any account of desire for trans people must be able to see trans people as desirable. In other words, accounts that uniformly treat desire for trans people as constituting a fetish serve to deny the desirability of trans people. Certainly, fetishising is an issue faced by some trans people, as we explored in the previous section. But, as Tompkins argues, reducing all desire for trans people by cisgender people to a fetish denies the possibility of a sex-positive account of trans people's intimate lives.

So too, Edelman and Zimman (2014) argue that an over focus on dysphoria serves to minimise the desires that trans people experience, and also serves to position trans people as undesirable. By contrast, Edelman and Zimman argue that in encounters between trans masculine people and cisgender men, trans masculine people's bodies may be seen as desirable. As they argue, trans masculine people negotiate norms of masculine embodiment, specifically by naming their bodies in ways that position their bodies as masculine, and hence desirable to other men. Further trans masculine people may emphasise that, in addition to their bodies being traditionally masculine (i.e, by referring to a clitoris as a dick), trans masculine people may also frame their bodies (and specifically the vagina) as a desirable aspect of their body (i.e., in the language of 'bonus hole'). Edelman (2015) does question how, in doing so, trans masculine people may adhere to neoliberal discourses that require people to market their bodies as attractive to other people, but at the same time suggests that, by doing so, trans masculine people are able to negotiate desire and intimacy within homoerotic spaces.

Having considered pleasure and desire as aspects of sexual justice for trans people, we now turn to consider reproductive justice, and specifically areas that are often left outside of the more common discussions about reproductive justice for trans people that we discussed previously in this chapter. The first of these areas pertains to the menstrual needs of trans people. Lowik (2020) argues that the relative lack of attention to bodies that bleed other than those of cisgender women means that trans people's experiences are ignored, constituting a key aspect of reproductive justice requiring ongoing attention. Lowik highlights that for some trans people who menstruate specifically, journeys through, beyond, and involving the recommencement of bleeding (following the cessation of hormone therapy), highlight aspects of menstruation that evoke a sense of trans temporality: the idea that for some trans people the timing and passage of time related to gendered embodiment is uniquely shaped by cisgenderist expectations (Amin, 2014). Lowik further highlights that menstruation should not be viewed as limited to bleeding. As one of Lowik's participants noted, for some trans women monthly cycles are experienced, suggesting the importance of including trans women in discussions about menstruation.

Further, with regard to reproductive justice, Lowik (2017) has also been a strong advocate for the needs of trans people with regard to abortion. Lowik highlights how abortion services that continue to serve only cisgender women typically fail to create a space into which trans people feel welcomed, constituting a significant barrier to abortion care and thus the enactment of reproductive rights. Romero (2020) too argues that trans activism and abortion activism, while traditionally seen as separate spheres, can usefully be brought into conversation with one another. In part this is due to the fact that some trans people (or their partners) require abortion services. But more broadly, trans activism and abortion activism both centre rights to self-determination in terms of reproduction, and thus both have much to say jointly about how bodies are regulated. Seeing the two as separate repeats the idea both that reproductive rights are a private matter, and also that this fails to conceptualise a broader, public, political understanding of reproductive health that adds social flesh to how we think about bodies: both those of individuals and those of institutions.

Diversity in trans reproductive and sexual justice

Thus far in this chapter we have largely provided a relatively generic account of trans reproductive and sexual justice. To a certain extent, this is justified by the fact that many of the core issues – pathologisation, medicalisation, cisgenderism, and marginalisation – are evident across multiple contexts. Yet as we have indicated at key junctures throughout this chapter, in certain areas aspects of reproductive and sexual justice are context specific. As such, in this section we highlight some areas of both geographic and temporal specificity that require ongoing attention in any account of trans reproductive and sexual justice. In other words, while there are many similarities across contexts, some of the specificities provide unique needs for trans people.

In terms of reproductive health specifically, researchers continue to highlight differences in rights and access in terms of gender transition. Mendieta and Vidal-Ortiz (2020), for example, highlight that while Argentina has some of the most progressive (and the first) gender recognition laws in the world, in practice the implantation of reproductive rights has been less than forthcoming, especially in regard to access to abortion services. In the French context, Fiorilli (2019) argues that while laws have changed so that sterilisation is no longer required in order to affirm one's gender, the ultimate decision is still at the discretion of judges, who may still decide that an individual has not met requirements that allow them to claim membership of a particular gender. This echoes broader historical accounts of both medical transition for and gender recognition of trans people (Riggs et al., 2019). On the one hand, medical practitioners in the French context often resisted performing gender affirming surgeries on trans people under the guise of not harming otherwise 'healthy tissue'. But on the other hand, French courts have until relatively recently refused fertility preservation for trans people. Here, there is a tension between refusing treatment based on assumptions about 'bodily integrity', and refusing access to treatments that would ensure reproductive integrity.

Further, with regard to fertility preservation, in the Finnish context, while social health care provides for medical treatment for trans people, the law still retains a requirement of sterilisation in order for gender recognition to occur (Honkasalo, 2018). This tying of recognition to sterilisation thus provides a serious impediment to reproductive justice. In the Swedish context, laws requiring sterilisation have been removed, but as Erbenius and Gunnarsson Payne (2018) note, even after these changes occurred, and similar to the French context, judges authorising gender recognition could still raise questions about sterilisation, particularly with regard to stored gametes. As Erbenius and Gunnarsson Payne argue, this reflects a broader logic whereby reproduction is ideologically limited to cisgender people, meaning that trans people who reproduce are often framed as a threat to the body politic. Baars (2019) further outlines a number of international cases with regard to pregnancy that demonstrate how reproduction for trans people is positioned as problematic in terms of the body politic. In Germany, for example, a man who gave birth petitioned the courts to be recognised as the child's father, only for the courts, even after successive appeals, to refuse to recognise him as the father. Instead, the courts upheld the belief that all people who give birth are the child's mother, thus demonstrating how trans people's reproductive decisions continue in some contexts to be arbitrated by the state. In the United Kingdom, the same was true for Freddy McConnell, with the High Court upholding a decision that he could not be recognised as father to the child he gave birth to (Pearce, 2019). In the Israeli context, a trans man who gave birth and who had previously received legal gender recognition was required to change his gender marker so that he could be registered as his child's mother, only to have to change it again to then be recognised as his child's father (Baars, 2019). This type of administrative requirement demonstrates the types of reproductive oversight to which many trans people continue to be subjected.

Turning to consider sexual justice, and with regard to gender recognition specifically, there are at least 20 countries that do not have gender recognition laws (Transgender Europe, 2019). The lack of such laws has serious implications for the protection of trans people in general, but specifically with regard to sexual justice. At the institutional level, a law of gender recognition laws signals to society more broadly that trans people are not deserving of legal recognition and protection. At the individual level, not having documentation that accurately reflects one's gender can negatively impact interpersonal relationships, including providing a mechanism for coercive control in the context of intimate relationships. Even in countries where gender recognition is provided, however, this does not automatically translate into safety, including with regard to intimacy. Transgender Europe (2020) maintains a database of the murders of trans people across the globe, highlighting that trans women of colour are especially targeted. This targeting occurs both in public spaces, but also in private spaces, where trans women are met with sexual violence including murder by intimate partners. As such, while legislation providing gender recognition is important, it does not ensure safety, including sexual justice, given the ongoing effects of cisgenderism upon the attitudes of other people.

Finally, already in this chapter we have hinted at historical differences in terms of the reproductive and sexual rights of trans people. We have noted historical shifts and continuities in terms of medicalisation, pathologisation, desexualisation, and hypersexualisation, and the shifting terrain of laws protecting trans people. From the perspective of citizenship, the positioning of trans people's reproductive and sexual rights has long been framed through the lens of citizenship. As Serlin (1995) notes, for Christine Jorgensen, a trans woman who achieved notoriety in the United States in the 1950s, media representations repeatedly aligned her with her history of military service, positioning her as akin to a 'wounded soldier' who had given service to her country, and was thus deserving of care by the state. While this narrative of Jorgensen shifted over time, her inculcation within the body politic through tropes of war and damage highlight the investment in the state in rendering her as an intelligible citizen. Yet, this stands in contrast to other women –

specifically those who were not white, who did not undertake military service, and who were not feted by the media – who were not accorded a place within the body politic, and who were instead relegated to the margins (Snorton, 2017). This highlights the fact that while trans people have always been relegated to the margins, access to the mainstream – and thus to rights and protection – has always been further reserved for very specific groups of trans people, echoing our points earlier about transnormativity.

Our conceptual frameworks

In this section we outline the conceptual frameworks that we use in differing chapters of this book. These are in addition to the conceptual frameworks we have already outlined in this chapter. The first of these was reproductive and sexual justice, which focuses on the societal and institutional changes needed in order to ensure that reproductive and sexual rights can be enacted. Building on a reproductive and sexual justice approach, we have outlined previously Beasley and Bacchi's (2007) understanding of 'social flesh', which encourages a focus on 'thickening' our understanding of the relationship between individuals and institutions. Also previously in this chapter we have outlined the concept of cisgenderism, which is defined as 'the discriminatory ideology that delegitimises people's own designations of their genders and bodies' (Ansara & Hegarty, 2013, p. 162). Cisgenderism aids us in understanding the barriers that trans people face in enacting reproductive and sexual rights.

Intersectionality is another conceptual framework that we use throughout this book. First developed by Crenshaw (1991) to account for how women of colour experience multiple intersecting forms of marginalisation, intersectionality highlights the fact that aspects of our identity are not experienced in isolation. Someone is not, for example, black, and a woman, and a lesbian, with each additively resulting in an identity that is differentially marginalised. Rather, intersectionality emphasises that all three identity categories function simultaneously. Our earlier discussion of sexual violence against trans women of colour highlighted that such women experience violence resulting from the intersections of cisgenderism, sexism, racism, and colonialism. While much work using intersectionality has focused on people who experience multiple forms of marginalisation, more recent work has also focused on how intersectionality can help us understand the experiences of people who benefit from multiple forms of privilege, or who may experience both privilege and marginalisation (Riggs, 2010). In other words, using intersectionality to examine a diversity of experiences recognises that it is not only those who are marginalised who occupy intersectional identities. Rather, we all do. It is just that for some people systemic forces produce identities that are multiply marginalised, while for other people systemic forces produce identities that are multiply privileged, or a combination of both privilege and marginalisation. Importantly, this focus on diversity recognises that privilege is the corollary of marginalisation in the context of broader social forces where the former rests on enactments of the latter.

Feminist research is inherently critical (Hawkey & Ussher, 2022). Its starting point is the assumption that mainstream or traditional approaches to research have historically excluded or distorted the experiences of cisgender women and used male norms to define normality (Gavey, 1989; Grady, 1981). This includes the fact that differences between cisgender men and women have been historically construed as inferiorities on the part of cisgender women, with deleterious gendered implications for theory and practice (Martin, 1987; Ussher, 2006). The impact of social and cultural factors on women's lives has been negated, as have gendered power relations which are central to social life (Calder-Dawe & Gavey, 2019). In recent decades, attention has turned to the fact that 'woman' is often conceptualised as a unitary category, negating differences between women, and the intersection of identities – including ethnicity, sexuality, disability, and social class (Crenshaw, 1991). To account for the complex interlocking nature of these social identities, Patricia Hill Collins (1990) called for a paradigmatic shift of thinking by examining these identities within a 'matrix of domination' (Collins, 1990).

The phallocentric or patriarchal nature of research has also been criticised, with researchers accused of maintaining and reinforcing gendered power structures that negate the interests and needs of women and other marginalised groups (Stanley & Wise, 2013). This is ardently evident in distorted anatomical representations and understandings of cisgender women's bodies (e.g., the depiction of the clitoris as a diminutive penis) (Tuana, 2004) and through the development and testing of pharmaceutical treatment protocols that are skewed toward middle-aged, white males – seen as the 'universal standard' (Merkatz, 1998).

In recent years, feminist research has expanded to include a focus on inequality, moving beyond research on 'women' alone, described as "part of an evolving and developing political project that is not only anti-patriarchal but against all forms of abjection and abuse" (Harding, 2018, p.3). Feminist research is therefore applicable across a range of marginalised populations – including trans people (Johnson, 2015; Ussher et al., 2020). More specifically, a feminist intersectional perspective rejects unitary conceptualisations of 'woman', which are often based on a white, middle class, cisgender, heterosexual, and able-bodied ideal (Hawkey & Ussher, 2022). It is argued that theorists must consider the impact of more than a single identity or typical category of analysis to identify how the collective impact of simultaneous interacting identities shape power, inequality, and oppression (Bowleg, 2008; Hankivsky et al., 2010).

Another conceptual framework that we introduced briefly earlier in this chapter is that of trans temporality. As Amin (2014) notes, trans people's lives, like all people's lives, are marked by time. For trans people specifically, the operations of time may have unique effects, arising at least in part from the effects of cisgenderism. Young trans people, for example, may experience an acute sense of waiting for the future to start, given extensive waiting times to access services, and to be authorised to commence medical treatment. Trans people may experience a marked temporal shift between living as one gender, and living as another gender. This shift may be marked by the views of others, by societal narratives, and by an individual's lived sense of change across time. Narratives of time are common in trans people's autobiographies, used as a way to mark change. As Amin argues, such narratives of time both reflect an individual's lived experience, but also mark a dominant cultural narrative of trans lives (i.e., medical 'diagnoses' that mark gender transition by time, or the expectation that trans people either change or stay the same through the process of gender transition). The focus on trans temporality is thus both a focus on a very real phenomenon of temporal change, but also a culturally normative narrative about what it means to be trans, both of which are very much a product of cisgenderism.

Finally, in some of the chapters of this book we utilise the concept of 'gender euphoria' to counteract the dominant cultural narrative of 'gender dysphoria', and thus to put into practice Tuck's (2009) call for research that refuses damage-centred paradigms. Certainly, we do not mean here to refuse the very real experience that some trans people have of bodily dysphoria. Rather, our point here is that, just like narratives of change that produce a sense of trans temporality, narratives of dysphoria are treated as axiomatic to trans people's lives. 'Wrong body narratives' produce yet another form of transnormativity, one to which trans people are expected to adhere (Latham, 2019). A focus on euphoria, by contrast, celebrates the joys that trans people experience. As we explored earlier in this chapter, this may relate to joys produced through the agentic enactment of desire and pleasure. Euphoria may involve loving one's self or one's body (or parts of it). It may be produced through intimate relationships or through community engagement. Euphoria focuses on empowerment and agency in the face of cisgenderism, and indeed actively seeks to counter the effects of cisgenderism through a focus on joy and agency.

Chapter and project overviews and author positionality

Chapter 2 will explore how we understand pleasure, both within and beyond the context of sexuality, and the ways queer and trans perspectives on pleasure can inform concepts of pleasure more broadly. This chapter focuses on understanding how sexual pleasure interconnects with structural, interpersonal, and political issues that affect trans peoples' lives and wellbeing. The chapter develops a perspective of pleasure that underlies many of the proceeding chapters, particularly in the ways that trans peoples' access to pleasure is often denied, and the counteracting undertaken by many trans peoples in order to reclaim, subvert, and enhance pleasure and joy.

Chapter 3 will examine experiences and consequences of sexual violence for trans women. International research indicates that trans people experience a significantly increased risk of sexual violence, which includes both sexual harassment and sexual assault, compared to the cisgender population. Drawing on existing literature, and the findings of the Crossing the Line Study, a mixed method project involving in-depth interviews and photovoice, this chapter will explore the nature and impact of sexual violence against trans women of colour. Reports of racism combined with sexism, transphobia, and homophobia demonstrate the intersection of gender, sexuality, and cultural identity in trans women's experiences of sexual violence.

Chapter 4 examines experiences of sexual health care, as well as experiences of interactions with health care professionals (HCPs), in relation to the mental health and wellbeing of trans people, drawing on a survey of 699 trans people conducted in Australia, as well as published research in this sphere. We demonstrate that many trans people postpone sexual health care needs and avoid obtaining health care services due to their fears or previous experiences of stigmatisation, with a direct result on health outcomes. Mental health is better for individuals who are more comfortable discussing sexual health with HCPs. Equitable access to sexual health services is a human rights issue for trans people. Sexual and reproductive justice requires that trans people should feel safe and comfortable when seeking health care and should be treated with dignity and respect by clinicians.

Chapter 5 examines how Australian trans men construct and experience their desire for parenthood and through analysis of the experiences of 25 trans men who had experienced a gestational pregnancy. We argue that pregnancy can be a problematic but 'functional sacrifice'; however, formal assisted fertility experiences are rife with exclusion. Dysphoria associated with withdrawing from testosterone and the growing fecund body can be troubling, with changes to the chest of particular concern. Exclusion, isolation, and loneliness were the predominant features of trans men's experiences of gestational pregnancies. Health care systems are not generally supportive of trans bodies and identities and trans men encounter significant issues when interacting with health care providers. We argue that we need inclusive and specialised health services to support trans men through pregnancy.

Chapter 6 explores trans children's, young people's, and their parents' experiences and views on sexuality education and trans young people's reproductive futures, including fertility and fertility preservation. We argue that holistic sexuality education, which includes information relevant to the lives of trans children and young people, is important to their health and wellbeing and to the development of their sexual citizenship. Trans children and young people often make decisions about their future reproductive lives, relationships, family formations, and sexual health early in life. It is important that they are fully informed and able to discuss questions and concerns with knowledgeable parents, educators, and health professionals.

Chapter 7 reviews current knowledge about experiences of identity and embodiment for trans people with cancer and trans cancer carers, drawing on existing literature, as well as the findings of a project Jane has recently completed with colleagues entitled the *Out with Cancer Study*. As the chapter outlines, for trans people diagnosed with cancer, both the symptoms of cancer and the cancer treatment may affect gender, embodiment, and processes of gender affirmation. Further, the study identified heightened gender dysphoria and interrupted gender affirmation as the primary negative impacts of cancer on identity. However, for some trans individuals, cancer interventions had a positive impact, reflected in gender euphoria – comfort or joy in one's gender – and facilitation of gender affirmation. Interactions with health care professionals had the potential to exacerbate or ameliorate the negative impact of cancer on trans identity and embodiment.

Chapter 8 draws on two related projects undertaken by Damien and Clare Bartholomaeus. As two cisgender researchers, our interest in fertility preservation for trans young people stemmed from Damien's work as a psychotherapist, and in particular how he has witnessed trans young people navigating fertility services. Chapter 8 explores how trans young people and their parents navigate decisions about fertility preservation, and in so doing highlights how cisgenderism often appears to shape clinical interactions and the views of parents. Chapter 8 also applies the concept of trans temporality outlined above to explore how the passage of time holds particular meaning for trans young people navigating fertility services.

Chapter 9 draws on an international qualitative project developed by a team of researchers with a diversity of gender modalities and genders, comprised of Damien, Ruth Pearce, Carla Pfeffer, Francis Ray White, and led by Sally Hines. The project focuses on gestational parents who are men, trans masculine, or non-binary people, but also focuses on views about this diverse cohort of gestational parents. The specific aspect of the project that is the focus of Chapter 9 involved interviews and focus groups with young men, trans masculine, and non-binary people who were not parents, seeking their views on parenthood and reproduction. The chapter explores topics such as pronatalism, the prurient focus on trans reproduction often evident in society more broadly, and how participants view the relationship between masculinity and gestational parenthood.

References

Amin, K. (2014). Temporality. *Transgender Studies Quarterly*, *1*, 219–222.

Amin, K. (2018). Glands, eugenics, and rejuvenation in man into woman: A biopolitical genealogy of transsexuality. *Transgender Studies Quarterly*, *5*(4), 589–605.

Ansara, Y. G., & Hegarty, P. (2013). Misgendering in English language contexts: Applying non-cisgenderist methods to feminist research. *International Journal of Multiple Research Approaches*, *7*(2), 160–177.

Baars, G. (2019). Queer cases unmake gendered law, or, fucking law's gendering function. *Australian Feminist Law Journal*, *45*(1), 15–62.

Bauer, G. R., Hammond, R., Travers, R., Kaay, M., Hohenadel, K. M., & Boyce, M. (2009). "I don't think this is theoretical; this is our lives": How erasure impacts health care for transgender people. *Journal of the Association of Nurses in AIDS Care*, *20*(5), 348–361.

Beasley, C., & Bacchi, C. (2000). Citizen bodies: Embodying citizens – a feminist analysis. *International Feminist Journal of Politics*, *2*(3), 337–358.

Beasley, C., & Bacchi, C. (2007). Envisaging a new politics for an ethical future: Beyond trust, care and generosity – towards an ethic of social flesh. *Feminist Theory*, *8*(3), 279–298.

Bellweather, M. (2010). *Fucking trans women*. (Self-published).

Bowleg, L. (2008). When black + lesbian + woman ≠ black lesbian woman: The methodological challenges of qualitative and quantitative intersectionality research. *Sex Roles*, *59*(5), 312–325.

Brown, W. (2020). *States of injury: Power and freedom in late modernity*. Princeton, NJ: Princeton University Press.

Calder-Dawe, O., & Gavey, N. (2019). Feminism, Foucault, and Freire: A dynamic approach to sociocultural research. *Qualitative Psychology*, *6*(3), 216–231.

cárdenas, M. (2016). Pregnancy: Reproductive futures in trans of color feminism. *Transgender Studies Quarterly, 3*(1–2), 48–57.

Carter, K. J. (2006). The best interest test and child custody: Why transgender should not be a factor in custody determinations. *Health Matrix, 16,* 209–236.

Charter, R., Ussher, J. M., Perz, J., & Robinson, K. (2018). The transgender parent: Experiences and constructions of pregnancy and parenthood for transgender men in Australia. *International Journal of Transgenderism, 19*(1), 64–77.

Collins, P. H. (1990). Black feminist thought in the matrix of domination. In P. H. Collins (Ed.), *Black feminist thought: Knowledge, consciousness, and the politics of empowerment* (pp. 221–238). Boston, MA: Unwin Hyman.

Connolly, D., Hughes, X., & Berner, A. (2020). Barriers and facilitators to cervical cancer screening among transgender men and non-binary people with a cervix: A systematic narrative review. *Preventive Medicine, 135,* 106071–106071.

Crenshaw, K. (1991). Mapping the margins: Intersectionality, identity politics, and violence against women of color. *Stanford Law Review, 43*(6), 1241–1299.

Edelman, E. A. (2015). The cum shot: Trans men and visual economies of ejaculation. *Porn Studies, 2*(2–3), 150–160.

Edelman, E. A., & Zimman, L. (2014). Boycunts and bonus holes: Trans men's bodies, neoliberalism, and the sexual productivity of genitals. *Journal of Homosexuality, 61*(5), 673–690.

Erbenius, T., & Gunnarsson Payne, J. (2018). Unlearning cisnormativity in the clinic: Enacting transgender reproductive rights in everyday patient encounters. *Journal of International Women's Studies, 20*(1), 27–39.

Fiorilli, O. (2019). Reproductive injustice and the politics of trans future in France. *Transgender Studies Quarterly, 6*(4), 579–592.

Gavey, N. (1989). Feminist poststructuralism and discourse analysis: Contributions to feminist psychology. *Psychology of Women Quarterly, 13*(1), 459–475.

Gavey, N., & Schmidt, J. (2011). "Trauma of rape" discourse: A double-edged template for everyday understandings of the impact of rape?. *Violence Against Women, 17*(4), 433–456.

Gender GP. (2021a). Inclusive language and the menopause. Retrieved from www.gendergp.com/blog-menopause-inclusivity/

Gender GP. (2021b). Making cervical screening accessible for everyone. Retrieved from www.gendergp.com/blog-cervical-screening-access/

Grady, K. E. (1981). Sex bias in research design. *Psychology of Women Quarterly, 5*(4), 628–635.

Gruskin, S., Everhart, A., Olivia, D. F., Baral, S., Reisner, S. L., Kismödi, E., … & Ferguson, L. (2018). In transition: Ensuring the sexual and reproductive health and rights of transgender populations. A roundtable discussion. *Reproductive Health Matters, 26*(52), 21–22.

Gruskin, S., Yadav, V., Castellanos-Usigli, A., Khizanishvili, G., & Kismödi, E. (2019). Sexual health, sexual rights and sexual pleasure: Meaningfully engaging the perfect triangle. *Sexual and Reproductive Health Matters, 27*(1), 29–40.

Halberstam, J. J., (2005). *In a queer time and place: Transgender bodies, subcultural lives* (Vol. 3). New York: New York University Press.

Hankivsky, O., Cormier, R., & De Merich, D. (2009). *Intersectionality: Moving women's health research and policy forward.* Vancouver: Women's Health Research Network Vancouver.

Hankivsky, O., Reid, C., Cormier, R., Varcoe, C., Clark, N., Benoit, C., & Brotman, S. (2010). Exploring the promises of intersectionality for advancing women's health research. *International Journal for Equity in Health, 9*(1), 5.

Harding, N. (2018). Feminist methodologies. In C. Cassell, A. L. Cunliffe & G. Grandy (Eds.), *The Sage handbook of qualitative business and management research methods: History and traditions* (pp. 138–153). London: Sage.

Hawkey, A. J., & Ussher, J. M. (2022). Feminist research: Inequality, social change, and inter-sectionality. In U. Flick (Ed.), *The Sage handbook of qualitative research design* (pp. 175–193). Thousand Oaks, CA: Sage.

Hillier, L., Jones, T., Monagle, M., Overton, N., Gahan, L., Blackman, J., & Mitchell. A. (2010) *Writing themselves in 3: The third national study on the sexual health and wellbeing of same-sex attracted and gender questioning young people.* Melbourne: Australian Research Centre in Sex, Health and Society.

Honkasalo, J. (2018). Unfit for parenthood? Compulsory sterilization and transgender repro-ductive justice in Finland. *Journal of International Women's Studies, 20*(1), 40–52.

Johnson, A. H. (2015) Beyond inclusion: Thinking toward a transfeminist methodology. In V. Demos & M. Texler Segal (Eds.), *At the center: Feminism, social science and knowledge* (pp. 21–41). Bingley, UK: Emerald Publishers.

Latham, J. R. (2019). Axiomatic: Constituting 'transsexuality' and trans sexualities in medi-cine. *Sexualities, 22*(1–2), 13–30.

Lefebvre, D. (2020). Transgender women and the male gaze: Gender, the body, and the pres-sure to conform. Unpublished Masters thesis. University of Calgary.

Light, A., Wang, L.-F., Zeymo, A., & Gomez-Lobo, V. (2018). Family planning and contra-ception use in transgender men. *Contraception, 98*(4), 266–269.

Lindley, L., Anzani, A., & Galupo, M. P. (2020b). What constitutes sexual dissatisfaction for trans masculine and nonbinary individuals: A qualitative study. *Journal of Sex & Marital Therapy, 46*(7), 1–18.

Lindley, L., Anzani, A., Prunas, A., & Galupo, M. P. (2020a). Sexual satisfaction in trans mas-culine and nonbinary individuals: A qualitative investigation. *The Journal of Sex Research, 58*(2), 222–234.

Lowik, A. (2017). Trans-inclusive abortion services: A manual for providers on operational-izing trans-inclusive policies and practices in an abortion setting. Retrieved from https:// static1.squarespace.com/static/5cef632e66e9b80001f24e05/t/5d4115a2ec492200019f0c12/ 1564546469040/FQPN18-Manual-EN-PEI-web.pdf

Lowik, A. (2018). Reproducing eugenics, reproducing while trans: The state sterilization of trans people. *Journal of GLBT Family Studies, 14*(5), 425–445.

Lowik, A. (2020). "Just because I don't bleed, doesn't mean I don't go through it": Expanding knowledge on trans and nonbinary menstruators. *International Journal of Transgender Health, 22*, 112–125.

Mama, A. (2002). *Beyond the masks: Race, gender and subjectivity.* Routledge.

Martin, E. (1987). *The woman in the body.* Maidenhead, UK: Open University Press.

McKenzie-Mohr, S., & Lafrance, M. N. (Eds.). (2014). *Women voicing resistance: Discursive and narrative explorations.* New York: Routledge.

Mendieta, A., & Vidal-Ortiz, S. (2020). Administering gender: Trans men's sexual and repro-ductive challenges in Argentina. *International Journal of Transgender Health, 22*(4), 1–11.

Merkatz, R. B. (1998). Inclusion of women in clinical trials: A historical overview of sci-entific, ethical and legal issues. *Journal of Obstetric, Gynecologic & Neonatal Nursing, 27*(1), 78–84.

Obedin-Maliver, J., & Makadon, H. J. (2016). Transgender men and pregnancy. *Obstetric medicine, 9*(1), 4–8.

Pearce, R. (2018). *Understanding trans health: Discourse, power and possibility.* Bristol, UK: Policy Press.

Pearce, R. (2019). If a man gives birth, he's the father – the experiences of trans parents. *The Conversation*, September 26. https://theconversation.com/if-a-man-gives-birth-hes-the-father-the-experiences-of-trans-parents-124207?fbclid=IwAR1Anz8U_bgwiCPW1VNxpgABkawyfqmS98msx6tDzAQuRquxfze5YVjMK9k

Richardson, D. (2000). Constructing sexual citizenship: Theorizing sexual rights. *Critical Social Policy, 20*(1), 105–135.

Richardson, D. (2017). Rethinking sexual citizenship. *Sociology, 51*(2), 208–224.

Riggs, D. W. (2010). On accountability: Towards a white middle-class queer "post identity politics identity politics". *Ethnicities, 10*, 344–357.

Riggs, D. W., & Bartholomaeus, C. (2018). Transgender young people's narratives of intimacy and sexual health: Implications for sexuality education. *Sex Education, 18*, 376–390.

Riggs, D. W., & Bartholomaeus, C. (2019). Toward trans reproductive justice: A qualitative analysis of views on fertility preservation for Australian transgender and non-binary people. *Journal of Social Issues, 76*, 314–337.

Riggs, D. W., Pearce, R., Pfeffer, C., Hines, S., White, F., & Ruspini, E. (2019). Transnormativity in the psy disciplines: Constructing pathology in the *Diagnostic and Statistical Manual of Mental Disorders* and *Standards of Care. American Psychologist, 74*, 912–924.

Riggs, D. W., & Toone, K. (2017). Indigenous sistergirls' experiences of family and community. *Australian Social Work, 70*, 229–240.

Robinson, K. H. (2013) *Innocence, knowledge and the construction of childhood: The contradictory nature of sexuality and censorship in children's contemporary lives.* London: Routledge.

Robinson, K. H. (2022) Children's sexual citizenship. In Fischer, N., Westbrook, L., & Seidman, S. (Eds.) *Introducing the new sexualities studies* (4th ed., pp. 730–738). London: Routledge.

Robinson, K. H., Smith, E. & Davies, C. (2017). Responsibilities, tensions and ways forward: Parents' perspectives on children's sexuality education, *Sex Education, 17*(3), 333–347.

Romero, F. F. (2020). "We can conceive another history": Trans activism around abortion rights in Argentina. *International Journal of Transgender Health, 22*, 126–140.

Rosenberg, S., Tilley, P. M., & Morgan, J. (2019). "I couldn't imagine my life without it": Australian trans women's experiences of sexuality, intimacy, and gender-affirming hormone therapy. *Sexuality & Culture, 23*(3), 962–977.

Ross, L., & Solinger, R. (2017). *Reproductive justice: An introduction* (Vol. 1). Berkeley, CA: University of California Press.

Rydström, K. (2020). Degendering menstruation: Making trans menstruators matter. In C. Bobel, I. Winkler, B. Fahs, K. Hasson, E. Kissling & T. A. Roberts (Eds.), *The Palgrave handbook of critical menstruation studies* (pp. 945–960). London: Palgrave Macmillan.

Serano, J. (2007). *Whipping girl: A transsexual woman on sexism and the scapegoating of femininity.* Emery, CA: Seal Press.

Serlin, D. H. (1995). Christine Jorgensen and the cold war closet. *Radical History Review, 62*, 137–165.

Shannon, B. (2022). *Sex(uality) education for trans and gender diverse youth in Australia.* Cham, Switzerland: Palgrave Macmillan.

Snorton, C. R. (2017). *Black on both sides: A racial history of trans identity.* Minneapolis, MN: University of Minnesota Press.

Stanley, L., & Wise, S. (2013). Method, methodology and epistemology in feminist research processes. In L. Stanley (Ed.), *Feminist praxis: Research, theory and epistemology in feminist sociology* (pp. 20–60). London: Routledge.

Tolman, D. L., Bowman, C. P., & Fahs, B. (2014a). Sexuality and embodiment. In D. L. Tolman & L. M. Diamond (Eds.), *APA handbook of sexuality and psychology: Vol. 1. Person-based approaches* (pp. 759–804). Washington, DC: American Psychological Association.

Tolman, D. L., Bowman, C. P., & Fahs, B. (2014b). Sexuality and embodiment. In D. L. Tolman & L. M. Diamond (Eds.), *APA Handbook of sexuality and psychology: Vol. 1. Person-based approaches* (pp. 759–804). Washington, DC: American Psychological Association.

Tompkins, A. B. (2014). "There's no chasing involved": Cis/trans relationships, "tranny chasers", and the future of a sex-positive trans politics. *Journal of Homosexuality*, *61*(5), 766–780.

Transgender Europe. (2019). Trans rights Europe and Central Asia Map 2019. Retrieved from https://tgeu.org/wp-content/uploads/2019/05/MapB_TGEU2019.pdf

Transgender Europe. (2020). Trans murder monitoring. Retrieved from https://transrespect.org/en/map/trans-murder-monitoring/

Tuana, N. (2004). Coming to understand: Orgasm and the epistemology of ignorance. *Hypatia*, *19*(1), 194–232.

Tuck, E. (2009). Suspending damage: A letter to communities. *Harvard Educational Review*, *79*(3), 409–428.

Turner, B. S. (2001). The erosion of citizenship. *The British Journal of Sociology*, *52*(2), 189–209.

Ussher, J. M. (2006). *Managing the monstrous feminine: Regulating the reproductive body*. Routledge.

Ussher, J. M., Chrisler, J. C., & Perz, J. (2020a). *Routledge international handbook of women's sexual and reproductive health*. London: Routledge.

Ussher, J. M., Hawkey, A., Perz, J., Liamputtong, P., Marjadi, B., Schmied, V., ... Brook, E. (2020b). *Crossing the line: Lived experience of sexual violence among trans women of colour and those from culturally and linguistically diverse (CALD) communities in Australia*. Australia's National Research Organisation for Women's Safety.

Ussher, J. M., Hawkey, A., Perz, J., Liamputtong, P., Sekar, J., Marjadi, B., ... & Brook, E. (2022). Crossing boundaries and fetishization: Experiences of sexual violence for trans women of color. *Journal of Interpersonal Violence*, 37(5–6), NP3552–NP3584.

Vipond, E. (2015). Resisting transnormativity: Challenging the medicalization and regulation of trans bodies. *Theory in Action*, *8*(2), 21 44.

World Health Organization. (1994). *Report of the International Conference on Population and Development (Cairo, 5–13 September 1994)*. New York: United Nations.

World Health Organization. (2014). Reproductive health. Retrieved from www.wpro.who.int/topics/reproductive_health/en/

2

WHY PLEASURE?

Shoshana Rosenberg

> Yes, it is Bread we fight for – but we fight for Roses, too.
>
> *James Oppenheim (1911)*

When we think of pleasure, what are some of the most immediate associations we make? You may think of things such as chocolate, orgasms, or finding a corner in an 8000-piece jigsaw puzzle. But one other word that has been inevitably intertwined with pleasure is its pesky antecedent: *guilt*. What is the nature of this guilt, and where does it come from? The answers are myriad, interactive, and vary widely depending on each person's lived experiences and perspectives. You may place emphasis on structural issues such as fundamentalist religious doctrine, cisheteropatriarchy, white supremacy, or capitalism[1] as roots for our increasingly fraught relationship with pleasure. Or you may place emphasis on more personal experiences and learnings where your desires, whatever they may be, have been denigrated. The macro and the micro are of course perpetually enmeshed; each person carries cultural values within them which they enact, while also playing a role in either concretising or demolishing those cultural values.

Regardless of the machinations that lead one to the experience of guilty pleasure, the lesson learned here remains the same. We learn that wherever there is pleasure, guilt is surely just around the corner. Sometimes, heavy guilt or shame comes on in an instant, a visceral moment which radically shifts our relationship to that pleasure. A heavy, immediate wounding that leaves its indelible mark. At other times, however, guilt is formed through abstraction, expansion, mutation. Its seeds may be planted innocuously enough: a throwaway comment, a benign embarrassing event, or simply the total absence of open conversation about this or that source of pleasure. But the single cut left untreated soon opens wider, allowing more of these same small experiences through. Like an abscess in a pet's stomach, lying in wait to blow out your veterinary budget, the infection can grow slowly and go undetected

DOI: 10.4324/9781003138310-2

for weeks, months, years, a life. Without care, without covering these wounds in a healing and *pleasurable* dressing, we risk that guilt which has been foisted upon us making its way inside our bloodstream: inside *us*.

So why pleasure? Because this process of contamination, of turning things which gratify, fulfil, and delight into things which shame, repulse, and diminish, reveals the truth of how this illness can be combatted. Guilty and shame are toe tags placed on pleasure so that we may feel compelled to bury it. But in true horror fashion, despite the best efforts of oppressive forces,[2] *it's alive!* This is because pleasure is not simply an emotion or a set of actions which can be ignored, suppressed, or annihilated. Rather, it is a framework and worldview that is actively curative, sitting opposite guilt and shame by its very nature (brown, 2019). Pleasure grows like a weed, peeking through cracks and running wild wherever it is not being pruned or bombarded with herbicide. And like many so-called weeds, its persistence is only matched by its healing qualities.

We have been taught that pleasure is always verging on corruption, that it is constantly under threat. At any point, someone may catch you doing that thing which brings you such full body enjoyment, such pure bliss, and their words and actions will subvert or destroy your experience. This makes us guarded of pleasure, concealing and protecting it with increasing fervour the further we continue in the *guilt katamari* within which we are forced to exist. This can manifest in secrets, fetishes, complete and utter misery[3] … The consequences vary in scale and tone, but the processes through which guilt and shame are perpetuated are easily and consistently identifiable. At all times, it seems, the forces of the Guilt Nation press on deeper into Pleasurefolk territory. But this proverbial geopolitical conflict is a falsehood. Viewing pleasure as being on the back foot, as always needing to be defensive, denies the hope, power, and enormous growth it produces. It denies the tools forged by centuries of pleasurable human (and interspecies) interactions; the salves and ointments of loving words and actions refined between friends, lovers, families, and strangers over minutes, months, millennia; and the reality that guilt, like all other affects and emotions, is merely one force among many. Guilt is not invading pleasure, rather it is one player in a constantly shifting game of capture the flag.

Guilt triumphs through division, through isolation, through collective shaming and ostracisation. But pleasure's strategies to triumph truly represent its persistence in the face of these elements, its refusal to die off, and its determination to manifest itself again and again in even the harshest environments. Guilt is singular and fixed in its tenets and intentions; it is a suppressive force geared at de-energising, disassembling, or distorting experiences of pleasure which are liberatory or otherwise outside the confines of whatever dogmatic framework is being enforced. It is not always easy to detect or reliably identify, and its manifestations are many in both our daily lives and in the higher structures which (attempt to) govern them. Guilt and shame can be induced by someone yelling "faggot" at you from a moving car, by having your food consumption turned into a socially sanctioned moral failing, by living as a person in this world in any way which is seen as unwanted or dangerous. However, like guilt, pleasure also thrives on a diversity of tactics. It relies on deepening our relationship to our own senses, on physical and emotional connection with others, on giving body, mind, and community what they need wholly and unapologetically. Pleasure can be a late night cigarette, a first kiss, the feeling you get when you hear of the success and joys of others. It can be just as momentous and overwhelming or as subtle-yet-effective as any guilt-inducing experience or tactic. We are each in a lifelong process of attenuation between these two poles, of challenging, navigating, and overcoming guilt and shame, while at times fully capitulating into them.

If pleasure grows like a weed, then those of us who pursue it for its various qualities need to understand that "like weeds we will grow" (His Hero Is Gone, 1997). We are not separate from pleasure, and what we think, feel, say, and do about it either feeds or starves pleasure both in ourselves and in others. When we immerse ourselves in leisure, allow for unfettered indulgence, and squeeze every drop of opulence out of even the most fetid of materials and circumstances, we are both embiggening of and embiggened by pleasure. Pleasure is a pulsating, growing, multitudinous organism, at once a part of us and something with which we must actively engage in order to assure our mutual growth. This dovetails with adrienne maree brown's (2019) delineation of the personal, relational, and collective dimensions of pleasure; we need to internalise the knowledge that pleasure necessitates reciprocity, interdependence, and a forthcoming approach to inter- and intra-personal matters in order for us to experience it in its full glory.

So far the discussion of pleasure has been intentionally broad, as the subject is in and of itself one that holds many contradictions and controversies. In the proceeding sections I will discuss queer pleasure more specifically, and finally move on to explore how these frameworks of pleasure come together to form an understanding of trans pleasure specifically. It is vital that we comprehend the political aspects of pleasure as they affect us all, regardless of gender or sexuality. This is in part due to the kind of separation that often forms when discussing queer or trans issues, one where readers who do not fit into one or both categories may feel more like spectators than participants. Ultimately, the aim of this chapter is to expand our collective perspectives on how we interact with pleasure, and how gender and sexuality feed into these core human emotions and experiences, rather than siloing queer and trans perspectives on pleasure as something which resides solely in the realm of those of us with these lived experiences of so-called sexual or gender "difference".

Gay shame and queer pleasure

A preamble

Although I have been careful so far to include examples of pleasurable activities that exist outside sex, it is much harder to avoid the topics of sex and intimacy when discussing queer and trans pleasure. Ultimately, queer[4] people's Otherness is wholly defined by this point of difference; it is what has made us into curiosities, experimental specimens, and moral counterpoints which ensure our perpetually reinforced position as social pariahs (Greenberg, 2008; Stryker, 2009). From the moment that queerness began to be viewed as a social deviance that justifies violence, oppression, and criminalisation, queer people have used sex and pleasure as pillars of personal and public protest. This includes (in no particular order of controversiality): kiss-ins (DeLuca, 1999); barebacking (Crossley, 2004); public nudity (Schwartzwald, 1993); cruising (Shepard, 2009); the hanky code (Gellis, 2016); fisting (Stardust, 2014); being "out" as BDSM practitioners (Weiss, 2008); and myriad other pathways to penetrating the private–public membrane (Foucault, 1988), that which doubles as a thick veil separating the deviants from the pure-of-heart. In this sense, any discussion of queer pleasure must tread a certain balance, expanding the discussion beyond the realm of sex while acknowledging the power, beauty, and radical necessity of sex as a site of (queer) protest, connection, and indulgence.

It would also be disingenuous to discuss queer pleasure without acknowledging that there is no singular "queer" lens on pleasure. There is a documented history of queer people engaging in radically sex-negative actions extending now over several decades, with some prominent queer writers aligning themselves as proponents of certain levels of sexual "decency" or "normalcy" (Croce, 2015). And in the red corner, we have community members passionately defending their right to spit in their lover's mouth in a public setting (L., 2019), highlighting the deep, foundational, and ongoing history of Leatherfolks' and fetishists' involvement in the struggle for queer liberation (Baumann, 2019). In fact, it is precisely this point of division which leads us to consider the roles of pride, shame, and pleasure in the shaping of queer discourse and life.

Shame in Pride, pride in Shame

Where there is pleasure, we may uncover guilt; similarly, where there is pride, there is the leering spectre of shame. Over years of co-option and dilution, the public image of the "gay rights" movement has slowly but surely become sanitised by oppressive forces, shoehorning the expansive and diverse queer world into yet another seemingly legible box. This is nothing new, however; as Stephen Valocchi (Valocchi, 2017) suggests, structural forces (e.g., capitalism) have always shaped how queer people are (mis)understood and (mis)read by broader society. Historically and contemporarily, queer people have been sequestered to the realms of being *pitiable* and *wretched*; *mentally ill* or *degenerate*; *party boys* and *party girls*; *bringers of the apocalypse*; *vectors of disease*; the *shadow people* who are never spoken of; and (increasingly) people who are *"just like you, we promise!"*. But every attempt at ensnaring queerness under a singular term[5] brings with it sociocultural interpretations that determine how that community is regarded by broader society, and how the community regards itself. Therefore, before we unpack pride in Shame, we need to understand the shame in Pride.

In some ways, you need to look no further than any Pride parade in any major city to see some of the ways in which Gay Pride has catalysed Gay Shame.[6] Consider the increasing presence of corporations, banks, and cops at these events, not only as sponsors but as legitimate self-representing bodies with their own floats and adver-tisements. What is more shameful, more self-denigrating, than letting those who continue to oppress and kill us in through the front door? These are the same act-ing forces who turn affordable housing into parking lots; enforce foreclosures and debt collections on the most marginalised;[7] and assault, imprison, and kill queers and other marginalised peoples, respectively[8] (Mallory et al., 2015). Not only have many queer people welcomed this infiltration, but the presence of corporations and police has increasingly begun to enmesh with the broader queer imaginary (Russell, 2017).

Gay Shame is not legitimate shame, but a perspective that allows us to identify and uproot those aspects of ourselves and our communities that still induce shame and guilt under the guise of Pride. What joy do we achieve by approximating ourselves to our abusers and killers in the police force?[9] What indulgence do we get from seeing a Commonwealth Bank float full of grinning people who have already made more money than any one of us ever will? What opulence is there in an expensively made rainbow flag coat worn by a wealthy, white "gay ally"? These may be morsels for your eyes and ears, perhaps even for your soul, but this overi-dentification obscures the material reality of how these people and groups take away crumbs of pleasure directly from our mouths. You may like the gay cop on TV, or the limited edition Pride-themed bottle by whatever alcohol manufacturer feels most desperate for the "pink dollar" this fiscal quarter.

But these actors are not agents of pleasure, at their very core. They work to assimilate that which, fundamentally, could never be assimilated: the feral, opposi-tional, *pleasurable*, teeth-and-fingernails nature of being a faggot, a dyke, or a tranny. These forces attempt to control, "neaten up", and consequently *depleasure* queer and trans experiences. There cannot be a "faggot-identified" hedge fund manager, nor will we ever have a "dyke for president" (Leonard, 1992). There will be no Dr Tranny, Nobel Laureate. These are oxymorons, two north pole magnet facets being squeezed together indefinitely, and with ever-growing force. These notions of "order", "decency", and "success" have been foie gras'd into queer culture by forces whose mission is geared squarely at benefitting a few at the cost of the many, rewarding the elite for making the tallest staircase out of the bones, flesh, and debris of annihilated peoples, animals, and land. The systems, which create and dissem-inate those morsels of pleasure, are the same ones which strive to ensure that we will never have more than morsels. We are asked to suppress the very actions and experiences that bring us pleasure in exchange for a kind of public acceptance that is fragile at best and entirely false at worst.

There is no pride to be found here, not really. Like the delicate distinction between Leather and leather,[10] Politics and politics, semantics matter. Here, then, Pride is a brand, a logo which acts as both siren song and smokescreen. Pride™ intentionally aligns itself with one of the most collectively moving human emo-tions, the early battle cry of queers railing against their second-class citizenship and the oppressed lives that reality produces. To be proud of queerness is to be proud of survival, of how we fuck, of living a rich life through makeshift relational and geographic networks, carving out desire lines and forest clearings through stuffy thickets of straightness and cisgenderism. This is inspirational stuff, which has proven ripe for the picking to corporations[11] who have become wise to the marketing potential of these narratives. As with all things, though, capitalism and its proponents only benefit from a person, concept, or movement when they have been all but emptied of any sense of revolution, resistance, or refusal. Pride™ is a husk, a Potemkin village, relying entirely on its consumers buying what they are selling sight-unseen. Gay Pride™ is banks investing unknown amounts to create GAYTMs (Kaur, 2016) when many queers don't have enough money to make a withdrawal; gay pride is smashing those GAYTMs to smithereens (Mackley-Crump, 2018).

It is my intention to recouple politics and pleasure. Consider your own reactions to the two scenarios described above; which of these gets your blood pumping, makes your heart race, reinvigorates your sense of mischief and joy and power? More than likely, it is the one where we take some small revenge against corporate co-option and greed, even if that GAYTM gets fixed the very next day. Pleasure in so-called "visibility" is fleeting, temporary, superficial. But the pleasure of disrupting the supposed calm brought on by our acceptance (read: assimilation) into cisheteronormative society, of refusing those miserable crumbs from the banquet table, is something much more worthwhile.

Using shame

What then of shame? I'm wary of formulating yet another binary, one where we mustn't be prideful in order to be queer. I am not interested in negation as the only viable formulation of queerness; I reject our positioning as innately anti-(re)productive (Edelman, 2004). However, it speaks volumes to how queerness has become oriented in progressive discourse when we consider the totality in which *pride*, *outness*, and *integration* have been established as the fundamental pillars for a "good queer life". Each relies on the assumption that we must, should, could, and perhaps most importantly *desire to* share our queerness with the world. But if the ongoing rates of (predominantly Bla(c)k) trans women being murdered or queers attempting and completing suicide across all ages are anything to go by, these tools are insufficient in bringing about queer thriving and liberation.

Here, then, shame provides a fascinating counterbalance. So far I have discussed pride as a positive human aspect, but as with all aspects, the reality is much muddier. Pride also produces hubris, individualism, stubbornness, nationalism; ultimately varying forms and intensities of violence. We've had that figured out for a while now (Dyson, 2006). By contrast, if BDSM and Leather cultures over the last several decades have taught us anything, it's that some of the most seemingly painful things a person can endure are sometimes also some of the most pleasurable and worthy of pursuit. I argue that if pride receives a pass despite its shadow side, then perhaps shame should receive a similar treatment. In the same way that we must ask ourselves "what is pride concealing?", we must also ask "what is shame revealing?"

When we feel shame, we may shrink, become paralysed, attempt to flee, or buckle (seemingly helplessly) against its hold on us. This is the dominant narrative of shame, one where a shamed person becomes minimised, threatened, and dispossessed. Shame is thus made repulsive, only dealt with through counteraction, by pre-emptively minimising its place in our consciousness before it can minimise us. This battle is fought with what we perceive to be our full artillery: therapy, drugs, work ... We have become oriented to view shame as the opposite of safety, as a vicious creature that must be buried in concrete, staked in the heart, or beheaded, lest it rise again.

We have certainly got one part of this tale correct: it will rise again! In fact very little introspection is needed to recognise that shame, like all other emotions and affects, touches our everyday existence. No matter how productive your last conscious encounter with shame felt, no matter how cinematic and brutal the final scene seemed, it will rise from the grave[12] after the credits. So how do we contend with this recurring character? What are we missing from the armoury? Do we even need one?

It once again becomes pertinent for us to consider some of the perspectives that Leatherfolk and other BDSM practitioners have disseminated and refined for decades now. Specifically, we need to consider the deeply pleasurable aspects inherent within shame, and the ways shame facilitates, rather than negates, relationality and growth. Shame is not simply something that is being foisted upon us; it is also a unique tool that produces heightened emotional states that are rarely matched in their connection to power, control, and social status (Kali, 2017). Most people will find themselves unwilling or unsure of how to take hold of shame. In fact, you[13] may have never considered having an active, agentic relationship to shame, one which isn't simply a matter of withstanding its impact. But each of us is already holding the reins of shame, whether with feather-light touch or a white-knuckle grip. Certain aspects of BDSM have now fully arrived within the mainstream,[14] in particular those understandings of pain as pleasurable or perhaps even ecstatic, knowledge that perverts have been playing with since time immemorial (Bean, 1991, 1994; Brame, 2000).

While mainstream media and discourse provide a kind of semiotic depiction of consensual pain, and perhaps even consensual shaming, the emotionality and complexity are inevitably washed out in favour of shock value or humour. This too is an act of shame; transforming things which are abject or deeply uncomfortable into things which bring about relief. This forms a kind of shame ouroboros, one which cannot be untangled or fully understood in its current form. It is a self-contained story: there are things people do which are shameful, and we can look at them for a brief moment, but only in order to narratively alleviate that shame. At no point are we allowed to immerse ourselves openly in this *pleasurable shame* for more than a few moments, enough to move through the beats of the joke or to reach the underlying moral of the story being told. What we fail to understand is that this is exactly the mechanism through which we have been deprived of the productive power of shame.

Shame forms a critical tension between ourselves and the world. We must respect or at the very least accept the persistence of shame, because despite its many negative connotations it draws a distinct line in the sand which guides our way forward. Eric Stanley's (Stanley, 2018) consideration of the Left's obsession with positive emotionality and affects as the only throughfare is a reminder that our approach to pleasure can never be arbitrary, can never be reduced down to a set of words or actions that guarantee pleasure. After all, one person's depravity is another person's delight! Similarly, the point of pleasure is not that it is a gold standard to which we must strive, or an imperative that will make or break our capacity to integrate into the world (Lovelock, 2019). Rather, queer pleasure is a horizon (Muñoz et al., 2019) of possibilities and iterations of inner and outer relationships which we may feel compelled to swim towards.

Despite our collective aversion to facing shame head on, shame fuels many radical aspects of life. Politically, queer peoples' shame in gay assimilation has resulted in actions such as the Exploitation Runway (Stanley, 2018) or anti-police protests levelled at Mardi Gras organisers (Dwyer, 2014; Ellis, 2019). Relationally, collective queer shame is also often where we find each other, in the poorly lit corners and relational or geographical outskirts to which we are shamefully (self-)banished; even in our painful navigation of shame, we remain active actors who choose to touch hands in the dark and fuck who we want where we can. Which leads to the most crucial aspect at the core of all of this: *shame is hot.* We cannot separate shame's connection to fucking, to bodies touching (or not), to physical actions that mesh interpersonal similarities and differences together to form a mess of flesh and sweat and cum.

Fucking with (trans) bodies

I have been slowly building an argument that shame exists within our bodies, that it is a source of power we relate with daily, and that it is not as clearly delineated in its affect as we would like to believe. But we must move beyond a purely intellectual contemplation of shame as an inroad to pleasure. It is vital to recognise that this embodied moment of collision between shame and pleasure, this radical nexus, is a fountainhead of pleasurable insight. This point of transformation, the otherworldly ooze inside a *mariposa*'s chrysalis, is also what provides us with a bridge to the specificities of trans pleasure.

Trans narratives in the broader public discourse adhere fairly strictly to a kind of *mythos/leper* binary. We are either exquisitely pleasurable and borderline-supernatural creatures who colour the world with our mere presence, or we are the aforementioned archetypal pitied wretches of the world. In other words, we can only exist as abstract symbols of either pleasure or suffering. This disembodying and objectifying reduction is very telling, in that it reveals just how heavy the fog of war surrounding both gender and pleasure is, particularly for people who have not experienced the ecstasy of genderfucking, transsexualism, crossdressing, or any other means of accessing the gender/pleasure melting pot. Fortunately, no matter how many times this knowledge of the pleasure inherent to the experience of gender exploration and affirmation is both literally and discursively destroyed, our stories find their foothold.

Archives have been burnt (Bauer, 2014), storytellers have found their early and often tragic demise (Jackson, 2021), and government policies have only been further tightened to restrict our freedom to access these core pleasures (Latham, 2020; McArdle, 2016); and yet, people continue to define and redefine their gender outside of binary and cisgenderist societal expectations every single day. Ironically, bioessentialist claims around the 'truth' of bodies (in terms of claims that sex = gender, and that only two sexes exist) hold a kernel of legitimate truth, in that no matter how oppressive a community or culture is towards transness and other non-binary understandings of gender, a lightbulb goes on in the bodyminds of people every single day which signals a need to exist beyond those systems. Yes, bodies (and minds) *do* tell a story, and time and time again that story is one of departure, of difference, of a life beyond restrictive duality.

Opponents of trans rights and deniers of trans existence are doomed to contemplate the subject of bodies in only the most superficial terms, never going beyond the information found in the yellowed pages of biology textbooks and Spinifex Press manuscripts or the ramblings of others like them, whether at the pulpit, on Reddit, or in parliament. More heartbreaking is the implication this has for those folks who cling most strongly to these (somehow both shockingly new and heavily outdated) understandings of bodies and gender:[15] the gaps of self-knowledge that trans people must parse in order to self-actualise are left as yawning chasms of unknowing to those who are reticent to explore these understandings. Cisgenderism, at its core, is a self-limiting belief, as it requires one to avoid asking many crucial questions about their bodymind as it relates to both itself and to others. If a cisgender woman cannot question her sex, not just in terms of its positioning in society but in terms of its legitimacy as an axis of difference, how could she ever unshackle herself from the patriarchal system that preys on her wholesale acceptance of the 'truth' of men and women? If a cisgender man truly believes that certain hormones and chromosomes produce certain mindsets and behaviours, namely callousness and violence and dominance in his case, how could he possibly resist those actions and bring forth a better life for himself and those around him? In the realm of sexual pleasure, what chance do either of these subjects have to understand the plethora of joy and wonder and pleasant surprises which come from decoupling physiology from behavioural and attitudinal expectations and actions?

To say that cisgenderist framings of gender have a reductive effect on pleasure is an almost painful understatement. Take for example the orgasm gap (Mahar et al., 2020), a truly well-established understanding of the radical difference in levels of pleasure within cishet relationships, with cisgender men coming[16] out on top by a wide margin. Yes, it is a matter of patriarchal disregard for women's pleasure, often to the extent that bringing about this pleasure (through mechanical or clinical means) was seen as merely a treatment for their psychological distress (Maines, 2001). But it is also a matter of self-ignorance, one manufactured and carried forward by a system which positions male and female bodies as diametric opposites with restricted capacities and potentials. Sure, cisgender men may have more orgasms, but how much pleasure could possibly be gained by either party in the handful of minutes an average 'mixed sex' sexual encounter lasts (Blair & Pukall, 2014)? The dominance of the narrative of (cis male) penis in (cis female) vagina as the only legitimate sexual act narrows its proponents' scope of pleasurable experiences from a coursing river to a spittle. Even the notion of the orgasm gap itself is performed in front of the backdrop of cisgenderism and heterosexism, where genital climax is positioned as the singular landmark of a pleasurable sexual experience. There is no room in this rigid tale for indulging in silicone (Preciado, 2018), in leather (Bean, 1994), in penetrating non-vaginal/anal holes (Bellwether, 2013), in sex that is more to do with gendered becoming and unenveloping than rigid re-enactment of pre-existing gender narratives (Kaldera, 2009).

There is a well-worn idea that queerness and transness exist outside societal narratives (Warner, 2000), and that this outsideness is mostly if not wholly something negative, forcing each person to find resolution within themself in order to alleviate the tension (Halberstam & Halberstam, 2005). This idea that fitting oneself into templates brings about peace and quietude is not without its merits, but quickly loses power when one considers what is forfeited when we acquiesce to what already exists, rather than continually stretch ourselves towards that queer horizon. We have not arrived at our present queer moment(s) through conformity, nor will we thrive by settling for what has been achieved by others before us. There is a kind of rolling amnesia at play here, a perpetual forgetfulness of the energy and collective action required to keep the kind of momentum going that got queer people to where we are and has secured (some of) us (some) safety.

It can be hard for outsiders to comprehend the sheer generative force of transness in all its complexity. I specifically use the term 'generative' here to separate this term from any fairy tale of 'trans magic', for generation requires both construction and destruction, not the seemingly endless upwards growth implied by the proliferation of the notion of the 'trans tipping point' (Ryan, 2009). Healthy forests do not only require water, but fire too. Trans people must destroy, deconstruct, or heavy-handedly reshape many things in order to build ourselves: our families, our intrapersonal connections, our physical bodies. This includes coming face to face with many of society's most shameful facets just so we can make it through another day. We are confronted with the shame of disappointing family and friends, the shame of falling severely short of whatever feminine or masculine ideals have been foisted upon us, the shame of having our bodies exposed and touched and turned into discussion points or politicised hypotheticals in our attempts to receive even a crumb of humanity from the master's table. We are subjected to non-consensual genital examinations (Samuels et al., 2018), dehumanising political circuses based on the most banal of premises (e.g. trans people's participating in gender-segregated sports (Flores et al., 2020)), physical violence (Testa et al., 2012), and myriad other points of micro- and macro-aggressions which are directly targeted at inducing internalised shame (Stafford, 2012).

You need look no further than the Real Life Test (Levine, 2009), wherein trans people must live up to 12 months in their 'chosen gender' prior to receiving a medical diagnosis, a practice still perpetuated by many clinicians who work with trans people, to understand the shameful positioning of transness in the contemporary world. What could be more infantilising, more downplaying and degrading of one's own experience, than having to perform transness 'correctly' to a cisgender person just to access the basic needs of trans people seeking to medically transition or have their documentation reflect their gender? Not to mention the underlying implication that transness is something that must be *managed*, *observed*, and possibly *prevented*; it is positioned as a *disease process*.

And yet, we trudge on. We minimise ourselves at the right moments, flatten our narratives for societal digestibility, order our hormones illegally and access surgeries outside of our countries of residence, find comfort in kin when it is wholly unavailable elsewhere, whatever it takes to live as we need to. The processes described above may succeed in miserabilising us, for a moment or a lifetime, but they cannot take away the fact that we encounter shame daily and choose to cut off its head. Cisgenderist conceptions of pleasure might be accessible and ready-at-hand, but they also deny those devoted to them the rewards reaped through the undeniably hard labour required of trans people to experience even a sliver of pleasure in a world that wants us subdued and demoralised, if not entirely disappeared. Pleasure is a muscle, one that either atrophies through inaction or grows through intentional and directive work. When people are denied something as core to the human experience as joy, there is bound to be counteraction, no matter how small. It's one of the many ironies of trans existence, that being denied such principle aspects of humanity drives us *further* into the pursuit of fulfilment.

This is all not to say that such processes of oppression do not have a human cost, with mental illness and suicide attempts and completion remaining significant issues for trans people in Australia and elsewhere (Callander et al., 2019). However, for those of us who do survive, who do grow through the cracks, our understandings and experiences of life and its joys supersede both the cishet imaginary, and the material realities delineated by it, by a wide margin. Of course there are multiple ways into uncovering the deeper pleasures offered by the world, but even a cursory conversation with any trans person reveals just how much the experience of living openly in a transphobic society catalyses introspection, exploration, and investment in both the self and the other. It may begin as a matter of survival, but even the darkest roots can yield a dazzling bloom. We might feel galvanised to seek out community in order to access basic resources (e.g., hormones, doctor lists, housing), but inevitably we find so much more. We find others who reflect us to ourselves, or who embody things we couldn't even imagine a person could be. We find people who fuck and love radically, because every other aspect of their lives has already been radicalised. We find writings, recordings, performances, and spaces are only created and found through desperation, through back channels, through the kind of laborious investigation that can only be prompted by being pushed away from what is made available to the majority crowd.

Reading trans pleasure reparatively

It feels intimidating, almost irresponsible, to state that suffering produces pleasure, particularly when discussing the kind of suffering that has long-lasting if not terminal effects on those who experience it. At the same time, avoiding this topic risks becoming what Eve Sedgewick (Sedgwick, 2003) termed *paranoid reading*, where the grit and complexity of a person or community's narrative go minimised or undocumented in an attempt to paint a positive or uncontroversial picture of the subject. This happens most often with marginalised peoples who already experience negative and stigmatised societal narratives, and who have to carefully curate how they are depicted and understood by society at large in order to avoid further persecution and marginalisation. This niggling concern returns us to a previous point: we cannot be generative without risk, without movement, without extending ourselves forward and outward. In order to resist this *paranoia*, we must be *reparative* (Sedgwick, 2003) in our approach to trans narratives; that is to say, we must understand that necessity for richness and detail in our stories, not just the way it may or may not be interpreted by our oppressors. If I ask readers to denounce both the story of trans people as magical creatures (read: non- or super-human) *and* as eternal wretches (read: non- or sub-human), I have a duty to detail the nexus from which this narrational dichotomy emanates.

A paranoid reading of the previous section of this chapter might go as follows: "trans people experience incredible pleasures as a result of their marginalisation, and therefore any suffering they endure is balanced out by this enrichment". This reading might lead one to assume that trans suffering is justified by trans pleasure, a position many opponents of trans peoples' rights would delight in taking on. It produces inaction and apathy, if not outright derailment of the continued calls for improved living conditions for all trans people everywhere, under the guise of this supposed balance. But we are not willing martyrs, and the relationship between our pain and our pleasure is correlational, not causational. Trans people do not access deeper pleasures as a result of our lived experiences of adversity, but as a response, a means of reshaping our hardships in the same way we reshape our relationships, our bodies, our sources of income, and our lives as a whole. The access point to the pleasures discussed so far is not pain but personal and collective *growth* and *criticality*. These pleasures are not unique to trans people; we share our delights and insights with our cisgender comrades and accomplices, both intimately and communally. They would be the first to attest to this! We do not hoard this knowledge, nor do we assign it purely to trans peoples, but rather see transness as the kind of powerful and uncompromising existence that sheds light on the darkened corners of human existence as a whole.

I am personally divested from arguing for the uniquity of trans people, and instead view the experience of gender exploration, affirmation, genderfucking, and departure from the gender binary as the birth right of every single human being. Trans liberation does not come from 'inclusive' policies and 'pro-diversity' corporations: it comes from burning the entire thing down and starting again. I am not liberated until you are liberated, and neither one of us is liberated as long as we are denied our right to understand ourselves deeply, to consider the roles gender plays in our inner and relational worlds, and to embody these understandings without fear of violence and death. We cannot be reparative towards our collective understanding of trans people without also bringing into question the structures that perpetuate our oppression: white supremacy (Snorton, 2017), patriarchy (Lee et al., 2014), and capitalism (Cinicola, 2020), to name but a few. These structures, and those who benefit from their existence, pit us against each other along myriad axes, and only gain power when we lose sight of them in favour of focusing on our individual differences through the lenses they produce.

In reality, *none of us*[17] *lives a good life while burdened by the weight of these oppressive structures and institutions.* The concept of a matrix of oppression (Ferber et al., 2007), a means of assessing who among us is more structurally oppressed under certain conditions quickly diminishes in usefulness when we come to realise that many so-called facts of the world (e.g., rent, the gig economy, fossil fuel-based transportation) are produced either to directly reduce the quality of life for all human (and non-human) life, or in total apathy and disregard for those outcomes. Neither you nor I can experience true liberation as long as we exist in societies that minimise joy and maximise exploitation. There are many degrees of denigration, shades of suffering, and axes of adversity, and no two people, no matter how identical their belonging to this or that group, will have the same experience and outcomes as a result of those lived experiences. But we are all nonetheless oppressed, and have a lot of work left to do. Trans pleasure exists as a counterpoint to our own suffering, but this does not begin and end with our so-called acceptance or assimilation into this miserable post-colonial, late-stage capitalist world. It is direct resistance. If we are to temper the grief of our existence with celebration, we must ensure our banquet is big enough to feed everyone. If we are to party in the face of terror, we must ensure the dance floor is accessible to all. Trans pleasure is ultimately a matter of living abundantly in a world that is lacking, that takes away from us. Trans pleasure is acknowledging that there is enough here for us all.

Conclusion

This chapter explored how we construct pleasure, how we are systematically deprived of pleasure, and how we can re-engage with pleasure in ways that crush these tools of assimilation which have been weaponised against us all, whether we are queer or trans or none of the above. Queer and trans experiences of sexuality provide roadmaps to sustaining and revitalising pleasure in the face of directive destruction. Trans people in particular carry with us the recognition that the world is oriented against us, that we are afforded no place in it to even breathe, let alone cum. Yet, we persevere, not only in creating and expanding pleasure within our inner worlds, but in sharing that pleasure with others who are willing to listen. That, too, is an act of pleasure, if we allow it to be one; to listen to another's experience and allow it to permeate into our own understandings, perspectives, and lives; to revel in another's joy and contemplate the ways in which it might become our joy too. I hope these discussions may inspire you to explore your body's capacity for pleasure, to attend more closely to others' desires, or perhaps even just enjoy the feelings that come with reading a book chapter that mentions fisting, crossdressing, and the destruction of corporate property.

Notes

1 There are no wrong answers here.
2 Or angry villagers.
3 Though to the right person, all of these may fall entirely within the realm of pleasure!
4 Here used in the broadest sense of the term, in order to encompass the varying ways it is utilised in writing on both sexuality and gender.
5 *Including* the term "queer".
6 From here on the terminology shifts from "guilt" to "shame", as I expand the discussion towards both an external and forcibly internalised shame, as opposed to the largely inward-facing machinations of guilt.
7 Which often results in significant harm to those peoples' health, including the increased likelihood of suicidality (Downing, 2016; Mateo-Rodríguez et al., 2019).
8 Though often interchangeably.
9 Not to mention the wider heterosexual population.
10 The former being a description of BDSM, and specifically queer BDSM practice; the latter being the description of the material itself.
11 And other national and international institutions.
12 Or lake, or alternate demon universe.
13 Dear reader.
14 e. g., media such as Bonding, Billions, or Arrested Development.
15 e.g., TERFs, SWERFs, conservatives.
16 /cumming.
17 Bar a 'lucky' few.

References

Bauer, H. (2014). Burning sexual subjects: Books, homophobia and the Nazi destruction of the Institute of Sexual Science in Berlin. In *Book destruction from the medieval to the contemporary* (pp. 17–33). Berlin: Springer.

Baumann, J. (2019). *Love and resistance: Out of the closet into the stonewall era.* New York: W. W. Norton.

Bean, J. W. (1991). Magical masochist: A conversation with Fakir Musafar. In M. Thompson (Ed.), *Leatherfolk: Radical sex, people, politics, and practices* (pp. 303–319). Boston, MA: Alyson Publications.

Bean, J. W. (1994). *Leathersex: A guide for the curious outsider and the serious player.* Los Angeles, CA: Daedalus Publishing.

Bellwether, M. (2013). *Fucking trans women (issue# 0).* CreateSpace Independent Publishing Platform.

Blair, K. L., & Pukall, C. F. (2014). Can less be more? Comparing duration vs. frequency of sexual encounters in same-sex and mixed-sex relationships. *The Canadian Journal of Human Sexuality, 23*(2), 123–136.

Brame, G. G. (2000). *Come hither: A commonsense guide to kinky sex.* New York: Touchstone.

Brown, Adrienne Maree. (2019). *Pleasure activism: The politics of feeling good*. Oakland, CA: AK Press. Retrieved from www.booktopia.com.au/pleasure-activism-adrienne-maree-brown/ebook/9781849353274.html

Callander, D., Wiggins, J., Rosenberg, S., Cornelisse, V., Duck-Chong, E., Holt, M., & Cook, T. (2019). *The 2018 Australian trans and gender diverse sexual health survey: Report of findings*. Sydney, NSW: The Kirby Institute, University of New South Wales.

Chingy, L. (2019, June 17). Why kink, BDSM, and leather should be included at Pride. *Them*. Retrieved from www.them.us/story/kink-bdsm-leather-pride

Cinicola, P. M. (2020). Uncomfortable proxies in transgender minority stress research: An anthropological synthesis of transphobia. *Anthropology Senior Theses*. Paper 205.

Croce, M. (2015). Homonormative dynamics and the subversion of culture. *European Journal of Social Theory*, *18*(1), 3–20.

Crossley, M. L. (2004). Making sense of "barebacking": Gay men's narratives, unsafe sex and the "resistance habitus". *British Journal of Social Psychology*, *43*(2), 225–244.

DeLuca, K. M. (1999). Unruly arguments: The body rhetoric of earth first!, ACT UP, and Queer Nation. *Argumentation and Advocacy*, *36*(1), 9–21.

Downing, J. (2016). The health effects of the foreclosure crisis and unaffordable housing: A systematic review and explanation of evidence. *Social Science & Medicine*, *162*, 88–96.

Dwyer, A. (2014). Pleasures, perversities, and partnerships: The historical emergence of LGBT–police relationships. In D. Peterson & V. R. Panfil (Eds.), *Handbook of LGBT communities, crime, and justice* (pp. 149–164). New York: Springer.

Dyson, M. E. (2006). *Pride: The seven deadly sins*. Oxford: Oxford University Press.

Edelman, L. (2004). *No future: Queer theory and the death drive*. Durham, NC: Duke University Press.

Ellis, J. (2019). Renegotiating police legitimacy through amateur video and social media: Lessons from the police excessive force at the 2013 Sydney Gay and Lesbian Mardi Gras parade. *Current Issues in Criminal Justice*, *31*(3), 412–432.

Ferber, A. L., Herrera, A. O., & Samuels, D. R. (2007). The matrix of oppression and privilege: Theory and practice for the new millennium. *American Behavioral Scientist*, *51*(4), 516–531.

Flores, A. R., Haider-Markel, D. P., Lewis, D. C., Miller, P. R., Tadlock, B. L., & Taylor, J. K. (2020). Public attitudes about transgender participation in sports: The roles of gender, gender identity conformity, and sports fandom. *Sex Roles*, *83*(5), 382–398.

Foucault, M. (1988). *The history of sexuality: The use of pleasure*. New York: Vintage Books.

Gellis, B. S. (2016). Nature & spirit: A digital lens of gay-male culture. *Reconstruction: Studies in Contemporary Culture*, *16*(1), 4.

Greenberg, D. F. (2008). *The construction of homosexuality*. Chicago, IL: University of Chicago Press.

Halberstam, J. J., & Halberstam, J. (2005). *In a queer time and place: Transgender bodies, subcultural lives*. New York: New York University Press.

His Hero is Gone. (1997). *Like weeds*. Retrieved from www.youtube.com/watch?v=6GCCUveWL_I

Jackson, J. M. (2021). Black feminisms, queer feminisms, trans feminisms: Meditating on Pauli Murray, Shirley Chisholm, and Marsha P. Johnson against the erasure of history. In *The Routledge companion to black women's cultural histories* (pp. 284–294). New York: Routledge.

Kaldera, R. (2009). *Double edge: The intersections of transgender and BDSM*. Hubbardstone, MA: Alfred Press.

Kali, P. (2017). *Enough to make you blush: Exploring erotic humiliation workbook*. CreateSpace Independent Publishing Platform.

Kaur, H. (2016). *The determinants of consumer responses in the LGBT community: An exploratory study of LGBT marketing in the context of New Zealand and USA advertisements.* Canterbury, UK: University of Canterbury.

Latham, Hon M. (2020). *Education Legislation Amendment (Parental Rights) Bill 2020.* Parliament of New South Wales.

Lee, P. W., Lynch, I., & Clayton, M. (2014). *Your hate won't change us!: Resisting homophobic and transphobic violence as forms of patriarchal social control.* Cape Town: Triangle Project.

Leonard, Z. (1992). *I want a president* [Poem]. Retrieved from https://en.wikipedia.org/w/index.php?title=I_want_a_president&oldid=991484108

Levine, S. B. (2009). Real-life test experience: Recommendations for revisions to the standards of care of the world professional association for transgender health. *International Journal of Transgenderism, 11*(3), 186–193.

Lovelock, M. (2019). Gay and happy: (Proto-)homonormativity, emotion and popular culture. *Sexualities, 22*(4), 549–565.

Mackley-Crump, J. (2018). When a community stakeholder becomes alienated. *The Routledge Handbook of Festivals.* New York and London: Routledge.

Mahar, E. A., Mintz, L. B., & Akers, B. M. (2020). Orgasm equality: Scientific findings and societal implications. *Current Sexual Health Reports, 12*(1), 24–32.

Maines, R. P. (2001). *The technology of orgasm: "Hysteria," the vibrator, and women's sexual satisfaction.* Baltimore, MD: John Hopkins University Press.

Mallory, C., Hasenbush, A., & Sears, B. (2015). *Discrimination and harassment by law enforcement officers in the LGBT community.* Los Angeles, CA: The Williams Institute.

Mateo-Rodríguez, I., Miccoli, L., Daponte-Codina, A., Bolívar-Muñoz, J., Escudero-Espinosa, C., Fernández-Santaella, M. C., Vila-Castellar, J., Robles-Ortega, H., Mata-Martín, J. L., & Bernal-Solano, M. (2019). Risk of suicide in households threatened with eviction: The role of banks and social support. *BMC Public Health, 19*(1), 1250.

McArdle, D. (2016). Fear, loathing, and empty gestures: UK legislation on sport and the transgender participant. In S. Horlacher (Ed.), *Transgender and intersex: Theoretical, practical, and artistic perspectives* (pp. 67–81). New York: Palgrave Macmillan.

Muñoz, J. E., Chambers-Letson, J., Nyong'O, T., & Pellegrini, A. (2019). *Cruising Utopia, 10th anniversary edition: The then and there of queer futurity.* New York: New York University Press.

Oppenheim, J. (1911). Bread and roses. *The American Magazine, 73*(2), 214.

Preciado, P. B. (2018). *Countersexual manifesto.* New York: Columbia University Press.

Russell, E. K. (2017). A "fair cop": Queer histories, affect and police image work in Pride march. *Crime, Media, Culture, 13*(3), 277–293.

Ryan, J. R. (2009). *The transgender tipping point: It is not the transperson who is disordered but the society in which s/he lives* [conference presentation]. *International Foundation for Gender Education Conference*, Alexandria, Virginia. Retrieved from https://ai.eecs.umich.edu/people/conway/TS/IFGE2009/Joelle/The_Transgender_Tipping_Point.pdf

Samuels, E. A., Tape, C., Garber, N., Bowman, S., & Choo, E. K. (2018). "Sometimes you feel like the freak show": A qualitative assessment of emergency care experiences among transgender and gender-nonconforming patients. *Annals of Emergency Medicine, 71*(2), 170–182.

Schwartzwald, R. (1993). "Symbolic" homosexuality, "false feminine," and the problematics of identity in Québec. In M. Warner (Ed.), *Fear of a queer planet: Queer politics and social theory* (pp. 264–299). Minneapolis, MN: University of Minnesota Press.

Sedgwick, E. K. (2003). *Touching feeling.* Durham, NC: Duke University Press.

Shepard, B. (2009). *Queer political performance and protest.* New York: Routledge.

Snorton, C. R. (2017). *Black on both sides: A racial history of trans identity*. Minneapolis, MN: University of Minnesota Press.

Stafford, A. (2012). Departing shame: Feinberg and queer/transgender counter-cultural remembering. *Journal of Gender Studies, 21*(3), 301–312.

Stanley, E. (2018). The affective commons: Gay shame, queer hate, and other collective feelings. *GLQ: A Journal of Lesbian and Gay Studies, 24*(4), 489–508.

Stardust, Z. (2014). "Fisting is not permitted": Criminal intimacies, queer sexualities and feminist porn in the Australian legal context. *Porn Studies, 1*(3), 242–259.

Stryker, S. (2009). *Transgender history*. London: Hachette.

Testa, R. J., Sciacca, L. M., Wang, F., Hendricks, M. L., Goldblum, P., Bradford, J., & Bongar, B. (2012). Effects of violence on transgender people. *Professional Psychology: Research and Practice, 43*(5), 452.

Valocchi, S. (2017). Capitalisms and gay identities: Towards a capitalist theory of social movements. *Social Problems, 64*(2), 315–331.

Warner, M. (2000). *The trouble with normal: Sex, politics, and the ethics of queer life*. Cambridge, MA: Harvard University Press.

Weiss, M. (2008). Gay shame and BDSM pride: Neoliberalism, privacy, and sexual politics. *Radical History Review, 100*, 87–101.

3

VIOLATING BODILY BOUNDARIES

Sexual violence experiences of trans women

Jane M. Ussher, Alexandra J. Hawkey, Janette Perz and the Crossing the Line Study Team

Introduction

Sexual violence is a significant human rights and public health issue, with negative consequences for health and wellbeing (World Health Organization, 2013). International research indicates that trans people experience a significantly increased risk of sexual violence, which includes both sexual harassment and sexual assault, compared to the cisgender population (Blondeel et al., 2018; James et al., 2016). For example, a recent large-scale survey of trans and gender diverse Australians reported that 53.2% had experienced sexual assault compared to 13.3% of the broader Australian population (Callander et al., 2019). Similar rates have been reported in US-based studies (Stotzer, 2009). Trans individuals also experience high rates of verbal abuse and sexual harassment, which has been directly linked to their gender expression (Lombardi, Wilchins, Priesing, & Malouf, 2001; Ussher et al., 2022 a,b). In a recent Australian study, 72% of trans women reported verbal harassment and 79.8% sexual harassment in the last 12 months (Kerr, Fisher, & Jones, 2019), perceived to be associated with gender expression by the majority of trans women surveyed. The aim of this chapter is to examine experiences and consequences of sexual violence for trans women, drawing on existing literature, and the findings of the Crossing the Line Study, a mixed method project based at Western Sydney University, funded by Australia's National Research Organisation for Women's Safety (ANROWS).

Experiences of sexual violence are a significant contributing factor in the distress and mental health problems reported by trans people (Hawkey et al., 2021; Pitts, Smith, Mitchell, & Patel, 2006). For example, in the first trans mental health study conducted in Australia, Hyde and colleagues reported that trans people were four times more likely to experience depression, and 1.5 times more likely to experience anxiety disorders, compared to the cisgender population (Hyde et al., 2014).

DOI: 10.4324/9781003138310-3

Interpreted within a minority stress model, sexual violence compounds the chronic stress experienced by LGBTQ people as a result of stigmatisation and discrimination within a heterosexist and transphobic society (Cyrus, 2017; Hendricks & Testa, 2012).

Successive reports by the National Coalition of Anti-Violence Programs indicate that trans women experience sexual violence at rates significantly higher than all other groups in the broader US lesbian, gay, bisexual, transgender, queer (LGBTQ) community (2014, 2015, 2016). Trans individuals who are lesbian, gay, bisexual, or queer (LGBQ) may be further vulnerable to sexual assault or harassment on the basis of the intersection of gender and sexuality diversity (Callander et al., 2019). Trans women of colour, or those from a culturally and linguistically diverse (CALD) background, face discrimination and violence on the basis of the intersection of gender, sexuality, and racial identities. For example, it has been reported that in the United States trans people of colour are 2.5 times more likely to experience discrimination compared to cisgender people (National Coalition of Anti-Violence Programs, 2011). The largest transgender survey to date in the United States found lifetime prevalence rates of sexual violence at 45% for white participants, compared to 53% for black participants, 58% for Middle Eastern participants, 59% for multiracial and 65% for Indigenous participants (James et al., 2016). Sexual violence is often accompanied by other acts of physical violence, with trans people significantly more likely than cisgender people to experience physical violence (Dean et al., 2000). Trans women make up 8.6% of the LGBTQ community in the United States, but constitute 44% of total murder victims (Dean et al., 2000). The majority of trans women who are murdered are women of colour, poor women, or sex workers (Bettcher, 2014b), with many murder victims being all three categories. This has led to the plea to "centralise race and class as well as gender" (Bettcher, 2014b, p. 391) through an intersectional approach when attempting to understand violence against trans women. The remainder of this chapter will adopt this intersectional approach to examine the subjective experiences of sexual violence for trans women of colour living in Australia, drawing on existing literature, and the findings of the Crossing the Line Study.

"Crossing bodily boundaries": sexual violence experiences of trans women

The Crossing the Line study involved a survey of sexual violence experiences of 180 trans women, in comparison to 1249 cisgender heterosexual women and 866 cisgender lesbian, bisexual, or queer (LBQ) women (Ussher et al., 2020). We also conducted analysis of online posts about sexual violence experiences of trans women (Noack-Lundberg et al., 2020), and undertook in-depth interviews with 31 trans women of colour from CALD backgrounds, conducted by an interviewer who was herself a trans woman of colour (Hawkey et al., 2021; Ussher et al., 2022a, 2022b). The mean age of interview participants was 29 years (range 18–54 years). Participants described a range of gender identities, including "non-binary transfeminine", "genderfluid", "transgender female", "female", "sistergirl", "genderqueer", "woman", "trans woman", and "fa'afafine". Sexual identities included heterosexual or straight (29%), or gay, lesbian, queer, bisexual, pansexual, asexual, fluid (71%). Our interviewees defined their ethnicity as Malaysian, Aboriginal, Chinese, Samoan, Iranian, Indian, Tamil, Black, Sri Lankan, Filipino, Argentinian, Korean, Egyptian, or a combination of ethnicities. We adopted a feminist intersectionality theoretical framework (Crenshaw, 1989), that recognises that trans women are characterised simultaneously by multiple interconnected social categories, including gender, sexuality, social class, age, and ethnicity, and that these categories are properties of individuals in terms of their identities, as well as characteristics of social structures.

Rates of sexual violence: survey findings

Our comparative survey invited trans and cisgender women who had experienced sexual violence to tell us about the nature of this experience. The overwhelming majority of respondents indicated that they had experienced sexual harassment and over two-thirds of respondents reported that they had experienced a sexual assault since the age of 16, including trans women and cisgender women, across sexual identities and cultural backgrounds (Ussher et al., 2020). Trans women of colour reported more frequent sexual harassment than other women, with 70% having experienced sexual harassment ten or more times, compared to 40% of non-CALD trans women, and 56% of cis women. Strangers were the most common perpetrators of sexual harassment for all women, with trans women of colour reporting the highest rate of sexual harassment by a stranger (78%) compared to other groups of women (60% non-CALD trans women, and 70% cis women). Trans women of colour were also more likely to report being harassed outside the home or in public spaces than other women.

Whilst 50% of the CALD trans women who responded to the survey reported sexual assault since the age of 16, this was lower than non CALD trans women (66%) and cisgender women (66%). Though the majority of women who reported sexual assault had experienced it more than once, CALD trans women were found to be twice as likely as other groups of women to report having been assaulted ten or more times. CALD trans women were also more likely to report having been assaulted by a stranger and more likely to report being assaulted in the home and outside compared to other women. For further details of our survey findings and the methodology see (Ussher et al., 2020). We will now turn to the accounts of interview participants to examine subjective experiences of sexual violence, with pseudonyms allocated to maintain anonymity. We describe our participants as 'women', their preferred descriptor in the reporting of the research (Ussher et al., 2022a).

A hostile gaze and public mockery: "weird looks" and verbal abuse

The trans women of colour we interviewed reported that "sexual violence is everywhere", reflecting the high rates of sexual violence reported by trans women in previous research (James, 2016; National Coalition of Anti-Violence Programs, 2011; Sausa, Keatley, & Operario, 2007). It was during and after gender affirmation that the majority of our participants experienced both sexual harassment and assault, as reported previously (Levitt & Ippolito, 2014; Yavorsky & Sayer, 2013).

Sexual harassment was the most commonly reported experience. Every woman we interviewed gave accounts of feeling that they were an object of sexual interest and scrutiny on an everyday basis, manifested through "staring", "weird looks", or "disgusted looks". For the majority of women, staring was experienced as malevolent and described as "transphobic", as is evident in Lisa's account: "I've had a number of people stare at me before, as a trans woman. I think it [is because] this person is different sort of way. So, more transphobic rather than, 'Hey sexy'." Women who were openly wearing feminine clothes or make-up reported that staring was experienced as a violation, serving to "mentally undress" and make them feel "dirty". Gabriella's account illustrates this experience.

> They are all looking at me, because I was in a tight-fitting dress, so they're all trying to almost get this Superman X-ray vision to peek through my dress and see what is underneath, because always, when someone is mentally undressing you, I felt dirty.

In other instances, "looks" were unambiguously hostile. Sofia described waiting for the bus "and this guy walked pass me, he just gave me a look, a disgusted look towards me". She said that she thought, "This is so terrible that people have to throw their anger at you because you don't pass or you're just different". In each of these accounts, women are positioned as "other", as abnormal, through being the object of an inappropriate and invasive public gaze.

The majority of women we interviewed also described multiple experiences of overt verbal harassment by individual cisgender men or groups of men. Many incidents took the form of public mockery, which served to draw attention to and ridicule women's transgender status. This verbal abuse was derogatory and threatening, with women commonly being called "a faggot, a tranny faggot" (Jenny), "abomination" (Sefina), "pervert" (Sam), "shemale" (Petra), or "a freak" (Emma). This was experienced as an assault, as Sefina told us: "So, abomination, you're sin, what else? There's a lot. You know, weirdo, freak, 'Ah, you're a faggot, poofter'". These findings reflect accounts of verbal sexual harassment reported by trans women in previous research (Clements-Nolle, Marx, & Katz, 2006; Kerr et al., 2019; Xavier, 2000). This is a form of microinvalidation (Sue et al., 2007), the consequence of which was feeling objectified and hypersexualised, which could lead to fear, anxiety, social exclusion, or a situation of danger.

Many participants described verbal abuse when they attempted to use women's public toilets, being called "predators" or "perverts", invariably followed by attempts to exclude them. Jenny said that being questioned about her right to use women's public toilets is so common that she carries a letter with her to demonstrate that she is a woman, so if "somebody goes and complains that 'oh, there's this guy in the bathroom, in the toilet'" she can say, "Hey, listen. I might have something down there *but I am a female*. I'm going through the process of becoming a full female". Gabriella said that "people tend to overlook" the impact of verbal abuse on trans women, or tell women to "ignore it". However, this negates women's experiences, and the intention behind verbal abuse, to insult, intimidate, or threaten a trans woman because of her gender. This is what defined it as sexual violence, as Jennifer told us: "I think verbal abuse sexually, non-consenting, it's abusive". For Gabriella, and for many of the other women we interviewed, verbal abuse was positioned as an experience that was as "harmful" and "difficult to deal with", "if not worse" than physical violence. Indeed, verbal harassment often contained threats of physical or sexual assault, or acted as a precursor to physical or sexual assault. For example, Revathi was followed by men who said "they're gonna rape you and they're gonna − told me they wanna hit me, they wanna cut me, they'll throw me in the river".

Heterosexual men were the primary aggressors, for whom "taking on the feminine" can serve as deeply problematic to heterosexual masculinity, sometimes linked to the "taunt of homosexuality" (Yavorsky & Sayer, 2013, p. 154). This is evidence of the role of sexual violence in maintaining gendered power dynamics, and as a tool of patriarchal power. These accounts may be seen to reflect the objectification and gendered oppression of all women, with sexual violence grounded in misogyny and gender-based discrimination (Gavey, 2005; Langenderfer-Magruder, 2016). For trans women, misogyny is combined with transphobia, described as "transmisogyny" (Serano, 2007), with being trans and a women standing as multiple and intersecting risk factors for sexual violence.

Sometimes trans women were uncertain as to whether verbal harassment was sexist and directed at them as women, no different from "cat-calling" reported by cisgender women, or whether it was transphobic abuse because they "don't pass", as Lisa told us:

> It was a car that drove past me in the opposite direction, riding my bicycle. It was just a guy who gave a generic "woo" ... like a mean-ish scream towards me. Like, it wasn't any particular word, but, yeah. I don't know if it was because I was a woman or a trans woman who doesn't pass.

Such cat-calling could serve to validate femininity, as was the case when Gabriella was told by men she was beautiful, making her feel like the "prettiest girl in the world", illustrating the complex meaning of misogynist abuse for trans women (Levitt & Ippolito, 2014; Matsuzaka & Koch, 2019; Yavorsky & Sayer, 2013). However, many of the women we interviewed saw danger in "taking the compliment" as a man might "do something to her" if her trans identity is revealed. For if they were discovered to be trans through invasive touching or other forms of "genital verification" such as groping (Bettcher, 2014a, p. 394), this could serve to reinforce media representations of trans women as "sexualised deceivers" (Serano, 2007), precipitating physical sexual violence. For example, Jennifer explained:

I feel like if the guy is trying to hit on me and if they found out later on that I'm trans, they're going to be mad at me and my life is going to be in danger. For me, that's something that I always avoid.

In some instances, a woman being told she is "sexy" was overtly threatening. Mei gave an example of walking down the street, and a man coming close to her and suddenly saying, "You look very sexy". She said that "It's definitely sexual violence, because he didn't do any body activity to me, but the language is already doing the sexual violence".

Reports of racism combined with sexism and transphobia demonstrate the intersection of gender, sexuality, and cultural identity in trans women's experiences of verbal harassment, evidence of the "everyday racism" of "microaggressions" (Sue et al., 2007, p. 271). Many women of colour reported lifelong experiences of being subjected to verbal racist harassment, which compounded, or was a component of, their experience of verbal harassment as trans women. Natasha described her school experience as "just like shit in the playground like, 'Go back to where you came from'". Claudia said that she had a fair amount of body hair growing up" and as a result was "called gorilla a few times by some of the white boys". She also regularly experienced "casual racism" as an adult which was supposed to be a joke. She said "I don't find it funny". Jenny described herself and other Indigenous sister–girls being held in "the city watch house", the men's prison, in the late 1980s, and being subjected to racist and homophobic threats of sexual violence from male prisoners.

> They call us every name under the sun. They called us "faggots turn around" and threaten us saying "We're gonna rape you and fuck you up your fucking ass, you faggot!" "I'll fuck you up your ass!" and lovely things like that.

Jenny said that the police did nothing to stop this verbal abuse. Indigenous sister–girls may be more vulnerable to this form of ostracisation and verbal abuse, given the "over-policing" of Aboriginal communities in Australia, in particular, Aboriginal women (Cunneen, 2001). For other women, transphobia, homophobia, and racism were combined in online abuse. This is illustrated in Rena's account below, when she described men being "mean" and "harassing" her on online dating apps, then being "violent" in their comments if she didn't reply.

> Maybe they'll be like, "You fucking faggot", or "You're ugly anyway", and, "You – stop playing hard to get … you're not even a woman", or something like that …. This one guy he got really aggressive at me. He calls me a whore: #nevertrustanAsianwhore.

At the same time, a number of participants talked about experiencing transphobic and racist verbal abuse within the general LGBTQ community, sometimes from queer people of colour, as reported in previous research (Ellis, Bailey, & McNeil, 2015; Levitt & Ippolito, 2014).

Maya described how "narratives of violence" were often used against people of colour as a means to gate-keep involvement in the queer community, telling us it was a way to keep "trans people of colour out of spaces and to keep spaces as white as possible". This exclusion within queer communities serves to isolate "queer trans folk of colour" who need support, as Dinaz told us,

> Queers don't organise violent gangs to go round bashing people, but they do exclude people from communities which results in the death of people who no longer have access to their social networks or they feel like they can't rely on their community.

This is evidence of the othering of trans people within queer communities (Peters, 2018), which can result in trans women feeling marginalised or excluded (Bornstein, 1994), exacerbated by the failure of LGBQ support networks to address their issues and concerns (Crosby & Pitts, 2007). Compounding the direct impact of sexual violence, this provides further explanation for the high rates of distress reported in trans communities (Hyde et al., 2014).

"Crossing bodily boundaries": experiences of sexual assault

Appearing visibly different heightens the risk of violence for trans women, leading to the conclusion that the threat of sexual violence serves as "gender policing" (Jauk, 2013, p. 808). This form of gender policing impacts on all individuals who do not fit as expected within dominant norms of masculine/feminine behaviour as deemed appropriate to biological sex (Migdalek, 2014). This is amplified for trans women of colour who are simultaneously hypervisible as a trans woman and as a non-white person in a country dominated by constructions and impositions of cisgender white femininity in all areas of life (Graham, 2014). Staring and verbal abuse was often the precursor to physical sexual assault which served to "cross bodily boundaries", perpetrated by strangers, intimate partners, family members and clients during sex work. Many women saw this as a reflection of the fetishisation of trans women, which served to legitimate objectification and sexual assault.

Groping and unwanted sexual touching by strangers was a common occurrence for women we interviewed, with Mei saying, "sometimes a man, sometimes they will actually touch the woman's part". Many women described being frequently "groped" in bars or night clubs, as Maria said "half the time I've gone to bars I've been groped. I consider it harassment but apparently it's an assault thing". Being groped or touched on public transport, was also a common experience – including on buses, trains, or taxis. For example, Jennifer described a man "rubbing his dick on my butt ... then suddenly he grabbed my arse. The apparent social acceptability of this situation is illustrated by the response: "he just moved to a different place, and no one even tried to stop him".

Unwanted touch by strangers also took the form of rape or other forced sexual acts. Jenny told us that when she was looking for work at a country show, a man told her "If you come in the toilet with me and suck this, I'll get you a job at one of the sideshows. So, not knowing any better [I did it]". She said that as an adult "I've been raped quite a few times (by strangers)". Sexual assault was sometimes accompanied by physical assault. A large proportion of women described accounts of being spat on, slapped, hit, or stabbed. Maya described going to a party, "in heels and looking femme" when: "These guys just came up to me and they were all like, 'What the fuck is that?' And the one guy came up to me and just spat on my feet, like my heels".

The consequences of being perceived as gender nonconforming within a trans misogynistic and cis-normative society means conforming with sociocultural expectations of gender through "passing" is imperative for trans women (Miller & Grollman, 2015). Many women we interviewed reported being closeted, or endeavouring to "pass" as a cisgender woman in order to minimise the possibility of being identified as trans and as a result being subjected to sexual violence, as reported previously (Levitt & Ippolito, 2014). The majority of participants focused on being perceived publicly as a "normal" (cis) woman, with the "goal" being "just to pass, just to blend in". Jennifer said she was very happy because "any guy would just look at me, they wouldn't know that I'm trans". Passing meant that women were not in "danger" of transphobic verbal or physical assault, or being made to feel "unwelcome" in public spaces, as Jenny told us, "a person that passes, gets treated a lot better".

Not all trans women of colour could pass as a 'pretty girl' or 'beautiful woman' (Ussher, et al., 2022a). Dinaz said they could never pass because "I'm tall and I'm big and buxom", and as a result "I have to find the ways of being that are feminine but that also work with my body, not against it". Many women resisted or subverted ideals of white hetero-feminine beauty, which are "oppressive to women of colour with naturally 'frizzy hair'" (Deliovsky, 2008, p. 50), by embracing culturally appropriate clothes, jewellery, and hair styling (Ussher, et al., 2022a). Others who could not pass, or chose not to pass, embraced the "borderland" space in the middle (Peters, 2018). In embracing their gender and sexual diversity in ways they experienced to be culturally appropriate and valued, the women we interviewed demonstrated pride, agency, and resilience in the face of a world that was often hostile and exclusionary, through their intersecting gender, sexual, and cultural identities (Ussher et al., 2022a), as identified in previous research (de Vries, 2012; Singh, Hays, & Watson, 2011). Women also demonstrated agency in strategies they employed in an attempt to keep themselves safe from sexual violence both in the public and private contexts (Hawkey et al., 2021). Many participants described being "overly cautious" when in public and continually having to navigate a real threat of violence, as reported in previous research with trans people (Brumbaugh-Johnson & Hull, 2019; Yavorsky & Sayer, 2013). Others named sexual violence, sought out the positives in their experiences, and spoke to peers about their experiences of sexual violence – a topic that is frequently silenced in the LBGTQ community (Fernandez-Rouco, Fernandez-Fuertes, Carcedo, Lazaro-Visa, & Gomez-Perez, 2017). This evidence of agency, resilience, and resourcefulness has been found in previous research with trans women of colour who have experienced traumatic life events, including physical and sexual violence (Singh & McKleroy, 2011).

Danger in relationships: sexual violence within the family and intimate relationships

Many women were sexually assaulted by people known to them, and these assaults for some started at a young age, reflecting the established link between gender non-conformity and increased risk of childhood sexual abuse (Roberts, Rosario, Corliss, Koenen, & Austin, 2012; Walker, Hester, McPhee, & Patsios, 2021). For example, Sefina told us she was raped at the age of 12 by her cousin, who was 30. Although she felt at the time that "this doesn't feel right", she was also confused because the rape served as a "validation" of her feminine identity: "This man wanting me, and sexually advancing on me … attracted to me, to the woman". Amanda described sexual assault of trans women and girls as commonplace in Samoa. She said, "with boys, with men in the family, men in the village, you just shut up, toughen up and move on (because) they always expect that a fa'afafine is there to satisfy a male gender's needs". Many trans women of colour are subjected to sexual violence in the family (Cense, Stans, & Doorduin, 2017; Fernandez-Rouco, et al., 2017), with migration providing the only means to escape family violence and control. However, migration and the pursuit of asylum is a challenging process that can generate a new level of vulnerability and victimisation for trans women of colour (Alessi, Kahn, & Van Der Horn, 2017). Migration can bring resettlement challenges and experiences of racist exclusion and abuse (Alessi, 2016; Alessi, Kahn, Greenfield, Woolner, & Manning, 2020), with the intersection of cultural, sexual, and gender identities along with citizenship status increasing the risk of sexual victimisation for trans women during the migration process (Chávez, 2011).

Many women reported sexual violence in ongoing intimate relationships in adulthood, as reported in previous research with trans women (James, 2016). For example, in a study of trans women of colour in the United States, 44.7% reported intimate partner violence in the last year (Bukowski et al., 2019). Dating and the establishment of new relationships in adulthood brought a heightened risk of sexual violence, with many women being forced to undertake sexual acts, or being raped, on first dates. As Dora told us:

> I sat in the seat [of the car] and the doors were locked, immediately. It kind of turned into "if you don't perform oral sex on me I'm going to beat the shit out of you". My hair was really pulled, I got slapped in the face and I knew this was a very fucking bad situation.

Lin described despite only "planning to have lunch" with a date, things quickly escalated, when the man pressured them into performing sexual acts, "He was wanting to cum, I was just like – I don't really want to do this … he's like, 'Come on, come on'". Complexities surrounding disclosure of trans identity when beginning an intimate relationship with a cisgender man was associated with risk of violence. As Dinaz described:

> I think because a lot of people do want to hurt us … they feel guilty about finding us hot, they want to have sex with us but then they also have a lot of internalised homophobia, transphobia, a lot of cis straight dudes find trans women hot, and then they get the gay fear when they are engaged in sex.

Some participants talked about having to learn "that it's okay to say 'no' to sex" when they were dating. Lin had previously identified as a gay man, and said they had "just learned how to say 'yes' to everything because gay men are supposed to be super horny and you're just supposed to like it".

A number of women also described being coerced into sexual acts or "raped every night" within ongoing intimate relationships. For example, Elizabeth told us, "Over a period of time I kept on losing agency in terms of what I wanted". Sofia told us that she, "had a partner who was quite violent, like having sex and would not stop even though I asked [him] to stop". Although women could identify that their partners were sexually abusive, many said that they didn't feel that it was possible or easy to leave the relationship. As Amanda told us: "[I was] craving companionship, when you're lonely, [when] you're on drugs and you think no one else is going to be with you … [you] tolerate so much of the abuse … you learn to just accept it". These findings illustrate the particular vulnerability of trans women of colour who feel they cannot leave abusive relationships because of economic or psychological vulnerability (Moolchaem, Liamputtong, O'Halloran, & Muhamad, 2015).

"We face some violence from clients": sexual violence in the context of sex work

Sexual violence during sex work was common, including rape, physical assault, and men purposefully removing condoms without consent during sex, as reported in previous research with trans women (Lyons et al., 2017; Nemoto, Bödeker, & Iwamoto, 2011; Sausa, et al., 2007). Whilst some trans women engage in sex work because they have no other option in terms of making a living (Sausa, et al., 2007), others choose sex work because it is empowering, or culturally normative in trans communities (Fletcher, 2013; Sausa et al., 2007). Trans women of colour are more likely to engage in sex work due to having no other option, due to a combination of social disadvantage compounded by racism and transphobia (Weinberg, Shaver, & Williams, 1999). In describing sexual violence during sex work, Sefina told us "we face some violence from clients … hair pulling, scratches, punches came into play". Many participants reported that clients who would purposefully remove condoms without consent during sex, as Amanda told us, "You have the ones that forcefully, when you keep telling them, 'No, you've got to use a condom'… [and] they've trickily tried to pull it off, or they have pulled it off". Women also described experiencing clients who do "things that we didn't consent to" (Selvi), and if the woman attempted to refuse, this could result in intimidation and psychological abuse. Being a woman of colour could add to the risk of sexual violence during sex work, as Sasha told us: "Working in a brothel is safer and then the facts are trans women of colour are excluded from those establishments, so we are forced to work privately. Hence, we're more likely to experience sexual violence in our work".

Participants said they were rarely believed by authorities when they reported physical and sexual violence during sex work, and thus it went "unreported" and "unresolved". As Sefina told us, "People have said, 'Well you agreed to get paid', but at the same time, I didn't ask for a bloody nose, a broken eye, you know, half my hair pulled out." Selvi told us people have said to her, "Stop being a sex worker. You deserved it". Selvi went on to say that trans women of colour who are sex workers are frequently "powerless" to avoid violence as they often struggle to find other employment, resulting in significant financial insecurity.

> It is a problem for trans women because a lot of us may have difficulty finding work, so a lot of us look to sex work to make a living, at least in the interim while we're working things out and working up the confidence to even be able to be in public. It's such a common experience for us. So, yes, violence against sex work is a trans issue.

This is clear evidence of the intersection of social class, gender, and ethnicity in the vulnerability to sexual violence for trans women of colour who perform sex work.

Sexual violence towards trans sex workers is a serious health and human rights issue, which is associated with psychological distress, resulting in suicide attempts (Nemoto, et al., 2011) and substance abuse (Keuroghlian, Reisner, White, & Weiss, 2015; Sausa, et al., 2007). Trans women who were sex workers felt they were socially stigmatised and positioned by the police and within society as deserving of physical and sexual violence, as found in previous research with trans women sex workers (Fletcher, 2013) and sex buyers (Jovanovski & Tyler, 2018). Social stigmatisation is prevalent for all sex workers, but trans women of colour experience more social oppression and stigma than other sex workers (Weinberg et al., 1999). Our findings thus support Bettcher's argument that "the role of sex work must be seen as occupying a special role in our understanding of transphobia" (2014, p. 391). In contexts where sex work is heavily policed, or illegal, women are more vulnerable, highlighting the importance of the decriminalisation of sex work (Deering et al., 2014).

"We're turned into something we're not": fetishisation and the sexual "other"

Many women described feeling vulnerable to sexual violence because they were fetishised and positioned as "sex objects" or "exotic" due to their trans identity (Ussher, et al., 2022b). Jennifer told us: "One meaning of sexual violence for me, is to be objectified, because … guys make assumptions about what we are, and what we can do, we're being turned into something we're not". The concept, of being "different" or "mysterious" and thus of sexual interest was also evident in Dora's account where she said "in pornography … it's already kind of a fetish … having your own category". This objectification was associated with a feeling of lack of control in intimate relationships. Jennifer for example, discussed feeling as though she were a "doll". She said,

> People treat us as a doll, basically, they can do anything with it, they can remove clothes, they can dress us. A lot of people sees us as inanimate object … you don't have any control over what's being done to you. You don't ask a doll what kind of dress she wants.

Fetishisation could also be manifested as inappropriate questions or touching of women's genitals because they are trans, as Mei told us, "When you say you're a trans woman, they are interested in your original body parts, they say will it [penis] become smaller? This kind of uncomfortable words or uncomfortable actions, so they may touch it". Mei positioned this fetishised curiosity as "sexual violence".

Many women discussed fetishisation in relation to the intersecting nature of being a trans woman and a woman of colour, and the impact this had on how they were viewed by potential partners or sex work clients, primarily cisgender white men. Dora said, "There is definitely a thing about South East Asia, and trans women" and Elizabeth told us, "Asian women or South East Asian women are exoticised in the eyes of white men … there's that intersection of exoticising women of colour and also exoticising trans women". Women we interviewed positioned this intersection as contributing to higher rates of sexual violence and the dehumanisation of trans women of colour. For example, Maya explained, "Essentially, if you're fetishizing a person for anything, let alone the 'transness' or the 'brownness' … you're basically dehumanising them … [they] become the object of violence in that sense".

It has previously been argued that "non-trans people have a sense of entitlement about trans bodies … that warrants examination and study" (Fletcher, 2013, p. 68), reflected in the fetishisation and sexualisation of trans bodies (Ellis, Bailey, & McNeil, 2016). At the same time, the objectification and sexualisation of women of colour is central to colonisation and white privilege, reflected in cultural representations of African women as sexually lascivious and unrapeable (Watson, Robinson, Dispenza, & Nazari, 2012), and of Asian women as provocative, mysterious, yielding and vulnerable (Nemoto, 2006). In the present study, accounts of verbal harassment, bodily groping or assault, or being chosen by a partner or sex work buyer, were because of being a trans woman, a woman of colour, or both. Providing insight into the subjective experience of fetishisation of trans people (Ellis et al., 2016), these accounts demonstrate that trans women of colour are sexually objectified as a woman, a person of colour, a queer person, and a trans person. The intersection of these identities increases the risk of objectification and sexual violence for trans women of colour, and reinforces the importance of acknowledging the intersection of gender, race, sexuality, and social class when understanding violence against trans women (Bettcher, 2014a). The bodies of women of colour have been described as a space where racism, classism, and sexism converge (Watson et al., 2012). The bodies of trans women of colour are subjected to additional marginalisation, through the tyranny of transmisogyny.

Conclusion

The poor health outcomes experienced by many trans women are closely associated with their exposure to sexual violence and the social inequities and transphobia they are subjected to (Hyde et al., 2014; Moolchaem et al., 2015). However, the experiences and needs of trans women in relation to sexual violence remain poorly understood by many healthcare providers, legislators, the police, and policy makers (Smith et al., 2014). The absence of culturally competent information and knowledge about trans experience, accompanied by misinformation, can lead to stigma, prejudice, and discrimination, resulting in unmet needs for trans people. There needs to be recognition of the specific needs and experiences of trans women of colour, as well as education and training about gender and sexual diversity, to prevent sexual violence occurring. This must be accompanied by legislation and policy to address sexual violence experienced by trans women of colour, as well as other trans people, in order to provide protection and support. There is a need for education and outreach campaigns for both public and sexual violence frontline staff, including mental and clinical health professionals, and the police (Jefferson, Neilands, & Sevelius, 2013; Rymer & Cartei, 2015). This education should include ensuring trans women of colour are not victim blamed when reporting sexual violence and ensuring that policy, practice documents, and clinical guidelines use language that is gender and sexuality inclusive (Pallotta-Chiarolli, 2018).

Ensuring trans women of colour know about and are supported through the process of reporting sexual violence are also critical steps to address the significant underreporting of sexual crimes in this community. To ensure that policy and practice guidelines meet the needs of trans women of colour, it is critical that the voices of such multiply marginalised women are at the centre of leadership, program, and policy development (Battaglia, Edley, & Newsom, 2019), as identified by women who participated in this study. Policies need to challenge societal attitudes which support, condone, or trivialise sexual violence against all women, and recognise that trans women of colour and those from CALD backgrounds may need greater support from the healthcare and justice system when reporting incidents of sexual violence (Love et al., 2017). There is also a need for increased funding to establish sexual violence services that can employ staff who are culturally competent in supporting trans women, including the need to address co-occurring mental illnesses and facilitate women to efficiently process claims of sexual assault (Hawkey et al., 2021). Sexual violence is an urgent public health priority, in need of multidisciplinary, community driven, and culturally responsive measures that address the intersecting nature of discrimination, and inequalities experienced by trans women of colour.

Acknowledgements

The Crossing the Line Team includes the authors and: Pranee Liamputtong, Jessica Sekar; Brahm Marjadi, Virginia Schmied, Tinashe Dune, Eloise Brook, Kyja Noack-Lundberg, Samantha Ryan, Jack Thepsourinthone, and Rosie Charter. This work was supported by Australia's National Research Organisation for Women's Safety Limited (ANROWS). The views expressed in this paper are those of the authors and cannot be attributed to ANROWS. We thank the trans women who took part in this research for sharing their experiences with us.

References

Alessi, E. J. (2016). Resilience in sexual and gender minority forced migrants: A qualitative exploration. *Traumatology*, *22*(3), 203–213.

Alessi, E. J., Kahn, S., Greenfield, B., Woolner, L., & Manning, D. (2020). A qualitative exploration of the integration experiences of LGBTQ refugees who fled from the Middle East, North Africa, and Central and South Asia to Austria and the Netherlands. *Sexuality Research and Social Policy*, *17*(1), 13–26.

Alessi, E. J., Kahn, S., & Van Der Horn, R. (2017). A qualitative exploration of the premigration victimization experiences of sexual and gender minority refugees and asylees in the United States and Canada. *The Journal of Sex Research*, *54*(7), 936–948.

Battaglia, J. E., Edley, P. P., & Newsom, V. A. (2019). Intersectional feminisms and sexual violence in the era of Me Too, Trump, and Kavanaugh. *Women & Language*, *42*(1), 133–143.

Bettcher, T. M. (2014a). Trapped in the wrong theory: Rethinking trans oppression and resistance. *Signs*, *39*(2), 383.

Bettcher, T. M. (2014b). Trapped in the wrong theory: Rethinking trans oppression and resistance (Report). *Signs*, *39*(2), 383.

Blondeel, K., de Vasconcelos, S., García-Moreno, C., Stephenson, R., Temmerman, M., & Toskin, I. (2018). Violence motivated by perception of sexual orientation and gender identity: A systematic review. *World Health Organization*. *Bulletin of the World Health Organization*, *96*(1), 29–41.

Bornstein, K. (1994). *Gender outlaw: On men, women, and the rest of us*. New York: Routledge.

Brumbaugh-Johnson, S. M., & Hull, K. E. (2019). Coming out as transgender: Navigating the social implications of a transgender identity. *Journal of Homosexuality*, *66*(8), 1148–1177.

Bukowski, L. A., Hampton, M. C., Escobar-Viera, C. G., Sang, J. M., Chandler, C. J., Henderson, E., … Stall, R. D. (2019). Intimate partner violence and depression among black transgender women in the USA: The potential suppressive effect of perceived social support. *Journal of Urban Health*, *96*(5), 760–771.

Callander, D., Wiggins, J., Rosenberg, S., Cornelisse, V. J., Duck-Chong, E., Holt, M., … Cook, T. (2019). *The 2018 Australian trans and gender diverse sexual health survey: Report of findings*. Sydney, NSW: The Kirby Institute.

Cense, M., Stans, D. H., & Doorduin, T. (2017). Sexual victimisation of transgender people in the Netherlands: Prevalence, risk factors and health consequences. *Journal of Gender-Based Violence*, *2*, 235–252.

Chávez, K. R. (2011). Identifying the needs of LGBTQ immigrants and refugees in Southern Arizona. *Journal of Homosexuality*, *58*(2), 189–218.

Clements-Nolle, K., Marx, R., & Katz, M. (2006). Attempted suicide among transgender persons: the influence of gender-based discrimination and victimization. *Journal of Homosexuality*, *51*(3), 53–70.

Crenshaw, K. (1989). Demarginalizing the intersection of race and sex: A black feminist critique of antidiscrimination doctrine, feminist theory and antiracist politics. *University of Chicago Legal Forum, 140,* 139–167.

Crosby, R. A., & Pitts, N. L. (2007). Caught between different worlds: How transgendered women may be "forced" into risky sex. *The Journal of Sex Research, 44*(1), 43–48.

Cunneen, C. (2001). *Conflict, politics and crime: Aboriginal communities and the police.* Sydney: Allen & Unwin.

Cyrus, K. (2017). Multiple minorities as multiply marginalized: Applying the minority stress theory to LGBTQ people of color. *Journal of Gay and Lesbian Mental Health, 21*(3), 194–202.

de Vries, K. M. (2012). Intersectional identities and conceptions of the self: The experience of transgender people. *Symbolic Interactionism, 35*(1), 49–67.

Dean, L., Meyer, I. H., Robinson, K., Sell, R. L., Sember, R., Silenzio, V. M. B., … Tierney, R. (2000). Lesbian, gay, bisexual, and transgender health: Findings and concerns. *Journal of the Gay and Lesbian Medical Association, 4*(3), 101–151.

Deering, K. N., Amin, A., Shoveller, J., Nesbitt, A., Garcia-Moreno, C., Duff, P., … Shannon, K. (2014). A systematic review of the correlates of violence against sex workers. *American Journal of Public Health, 104*(5), e42–e54.

Deliovsky, K. (2008). Normative white femininity: Race, gender and the politics of beauty. *Atlantis, 33*(1), 48.

Ellis, S. J., Bailey, L., & McNeil, J. (2015). Trans people's experiences of mental health and gender identity services: A UK study. *Journal of Gay & Lesbian Mental Health, 19*(1), 4–20.

Ellis, S. J., Bailey, L., & McNeil, J. (2016). Transphobic victimisation and perceptions of future risk: A large-scale study of the experiences of trans people in the UK. *Psychology & Sexuality, 7*(3), 211–224.

Fernandez-Rouco, N., Fernandez-Fuertes, A. A., Carcedo, R. J., Lazaro-Visa, S., & Gomez-Perez, E. (2017). Sexual violence history and welfare in transgender people. *Journal of Interpersonal Violence, 32*(9), 2885–2907.

Fletcher, T. (2013). Trans sex workers: Negotiating sex, gender, and non-normative desire. In S. van de Meulen & E. M. Durisin (Eds.), *Selling sex: Experience, advocacy, and research on sex work in Canada* (pp. 65–73). Vancouver: UBC Press.

Gavey, N. (2005). *Just sex? The cultural scaffolding of rape.* London: Routledge.

Graham, L. F. (2014). Navigating community institutions: Black transgender women's experiences in schools, the criminal justice system, and churches. *Journal of Sexuality Research and Social Policy, 11*(4), 274–287.

Hawkey, A. J., Ussher, J. M., Liamputtong, P., Marjadi, B., Sekar, J. A., Perz, J., … Dune, T. (2021). Trans women's responses to sexual violence: Vigilance, resilience, and need for support. *Archives of Sexual Behavior, 50*(7), 3201–3222.

Hendricks, M., & Testa, R. (2012). A conceptual framework for clinical work with transgender and gender nonconforming clients: An adaptation of the Minority Stress Model. *Professional Psychology: Research and Practice, 43*(5), 460.

Hyde, Z., Doherty, M., Tilley, P., McCaul, K., Rooney, R., & Jancey, J. (2014). *The first Australian National Trans Mental Health Study: Summary of results.* School of Public Health, Curtin University, Perth, Australia.

James, S. E., Herman, J. L., Rankin, S., Keisling, M., Mottet, L., & Anafi, M. (2016). *The Report of the 2015 U.S. Transgender Survey.* In N. C. F. T. Equality (Ed.). Washington, DC.

Jauk, D. (2013). Gender violence revisited: Lessons from violent victimization of transgender identified individuals. *Sexualities, 16*(7), 807–825.

Jefferson, K., Neilands, T. B., & Sevelius, J. (2013). Transgender women of color: Discrimination and depression symptoms. *Ethnicity and Inequalities in Health and Social Care*, *6*(4), 121–136.

Jovanovski, N., & Tyler, M. (2018). "Bitch, you got what you deserved!": Violation and violence in sex buyer reviews of legal brothels. *Violence Against Women*, *24*(16), 1887–1908.

Kerr, L., Fisher, C., & Jones, T. (2019). *TRANScending discrimination in health & cancer care: A study of trans & gender diverse Australians*. ARCSHS Monograph Series No. 117. Melbourne: La Trobe University.

Keuroghlian, A. S., Reisner, S. L., White, J. M., & Weiss, R. D. (2015). Substance use and treatment of substance use disorders in a community sample of transgender adults. *Drug and Alcohol Dependence*, *152*, 139–146.

Langenderfer-Magruder, L., Walls, N. E., Kattari, S. K., Whitfield, D. L., & Ramos, D.. (2016). Sexual victimization and subsequent police reporting by gender identity among lesbian, gay, bisexual, transgender, and queer adults. *Violence and Victims*, *31*(2), 320–331.

Levitt, H. M., & Ippolito, M. R. (2014). Being transgender: Navigating minority stressors and developing authentic self-presentation. *Psychology of Women Quarterly*, *38*(1), 46–64.

Lombardi, E., Wilchins, R., Priesing, D., & Malouf, D. (2001). Gender violence: Transgender experiences with violence and discrimination. *Journal of Homosexuality*, *42*, 89–101.

Love, G., De Michele, G., Giakoumidaki, C., Sánchez, E. H., Lukera, M., & Cartei, V. (2017). Improving access to sexual violence support for marginalised individuals: Findings from the lesbian, gay, bisexual and trans★ and the black and minority ethnic communities. *Critical and Radical Social Work*, *5*(2), 163–179.

Lyons, T., Krüsi, A., Pierre, L., Kerr, T., Small, W., & Shannon, K. (2017). Negotiating violence in the context of transphobia and criminalization: The experiences of trans sex workers in Vancouver, Canada. *Qualitative Health Research*, *27*(2), 182–190.

Matsuzaka, S., & Koch, D. (2019). Trans feminine sexual violence experiences: The intersection of transphobia and misogyny. *Affilia*, *34*(1), 28–47.

Migdalek, J. (2014). *The embodied choreography of gender*. London: Routledge.

Miller, L. R., & Grollman, E. A. (2015). The social costs of gender nonconformity for transgender adults: Implications for discrimination and health. *Sociol Forum (Randolph N J)*, *30*(3), 809–831.

Moolchaem, P., Liamputtong, P., O'Halloran, P., & Muhamad, R. (2015). The lived experiences of transgender persons: A meta-synthesis. *Journal of Gay & Lesbian Social Services*, *27*, 143–171.

National Coalition of Anti-Violence Programs. (2011). *Hate violence against lesbian, gay, bisexual, transgender, queer, and HIV-affected communities in the United States*.

National Coalition of Anti-Violence Programs. (2014). *Lesbian, gay, bisexual, transgender, queer, and HIV-affected hate violence in 2014*. New York: National Coalition of Anti-Violence Programs.

National Coalition of Anti-Violence Programs. (2015). *Lesbian, gay, bisexual, transgender, queer, and HIV-affected hate violence in 2015*. New York: National Coalition of Anti-Violence Programs.

National Coalition of Anti-Violence Programs. (2016). *Lesbian, gay, bisexual, transgender, queer, and HIV-affected hate violence in 2016*. New York: National Coalition of Anti-Violence Programs.

Nemoto, K. (2006). Intimacy, desire, and the construction of self in relationships between Asian American women and White American men. *Journal of Asian American Studies*, *9*(1), 27–54.

Nemoto, T., Bödeker, B., & Iwamoto, M. (2011). Social support, exposure to violence and transphobia, and correlates of depression among male-to-female transgender women with a history of sex work. *American Journal of Public Health*, *101*(10), 1980.

Noack-Lundberg, K., Liamputtong, P., Marjadi, B., Ussher, J., Perz, J., Schmied, V., … Brook, E. (2020). Sexual violence and safety: The narratives of transwomen in online forums. *Culture, Health & Sexuality*, *22*(6), 646–659.

Pallotta-Chiarolli, M. (2018). *"Safe spaces, inclusive services": Support service access and engagement by LGBTIQ+ Muslims*. Melbourne: Muslim Collective.

Peters, J. (2018). *A feminist post-transsexual autoethnography: Challenging normative gender coercion*. London: Routledge.

Pitts, M., Smith, A., Mitchell, A., & Patel, S. (2006). *Private lives: A report on the health and wellbeing of GLBTI Australians*. Melbourne: Australian Research Centre in Sex, Health and Society, La Trobe University.

Roberts, A. L., Rosario, M., Corliss, H. L., Koenen, K. C., & Austin, S. B. (2012). Childhood gender nonconformity: A risk indicator for childhood abuse and posttraumatic stress in youth. *Pediatrics*, *129*(3), 410.

Rymer, S., & Cartei, V. (2015). Supporting transgender survivors of sexual violence: Learning from users' experiences. *Critical and Radical Social Work*, *3*(1), 155–164.

Sausa, L. A., Keatley, J., & Operario, D. (2007). Perceived risks and benefits of sex work among transgender women of color in San Francisco. *Archives of Sexual Behavior*, *36*(6), 768–777.

Serano, J. (2007). *Whipping girl: A transsexual woman on sexism and the scapegoating of femininity*. Emeryville, CA: Seal Press.

Singh, A. A., Hays, D. G., & Watson, L. S. (2011). Strength in the face of adversity: Resilience strategies of transgender individuals. *Journal of Counseling & Development*, *89*(1), 20–27.

Singh, A. A., & McKleroy, V. S. (2011). "Just getting out of bed is a revolutionary act": The resilience of transgender people of color who have survived traumatic life events. *Traumatology*, *17*(2), 34–44.

Smith, E., Jones, T., Ward, R., Dixon, J., Mitchell, A., & Hillier, L. (2014). *From blues to rainbows: The mental health and well-being of gender diverse and transgender young people in Australia*. Melbourne: Australian Research Centre in Sex, Health and Society.

Stotzer, R. L. (2009). Violence against transgender people: A review of United States data. *Aggression and Violent Behavior*, *14*(3), 170–179.

Sue, D. W., Capodilupo, C. M., Torino, G. C., Bucceri, J. M., Holder, A. M. B., Nadal, K. L., & Esquilin, M. (2007). Racial microaggressions in everyday life: Implications for clinical practice. *American Psychologist*, *62*(4), 271–286.

Ussher, J. M., Hawkey, A., Perz, J., Liamputtong, P., Marjadi, B., Schmied, V., … Brook, E. (2020). *Crossing the line: Lived experience of sexual violence among trans women of colour and those from culturally and linguistically diverse (CALD) communities in Australia*. Sydney: Australia's National Research Organisation for Women's Safety.

Ussher, J. M., Hawkey, A., Perz, J., Liamputtong, P., Sekar, J., Marjadi, B., … Brook, E. (2022a). Gender affirmation and social exclusion amongst trans women of color in Australia. *International Journal of Transgender Health*, *23*, 79–86

Ussher, J. M., Hawkey, A., Perz, J., Liamputtong, P., Sekar, J., Marjadi, B., … Brook, E. (2022b). Crossing boundaries and fetishization: Experiences of sexual violence for trans women of color. *Journal of Interpersonal Violence*, *37*(5–6), NP3552–NP3584.

Walker, S. J. L., Hester, M., McPhee, D., & Patsios, D. (2021). Rape, inequality and the criminal justice response in England: The importance of age and gender. *Criminology and Criminal Justice*, *21*, 3.

Watson, L. B., Robinson, D., Dispenza, F., & Nazari, N. (2012). African American women's sexual objectification experiences: A qualitative study. *Psychology of Women Quarterly*, *36*(4), 458–475.

Weinberg, M., Shaver, F., & Williams, C. (1999). Gendered sex work in the San Francisco tenderloin. *Archives of Sexual Behavior*, *28*(6), 503–521.

World Health Organization. (2013). *Global and regional estimates of violence against women: Prevalence and health effects of intimate partner violence and nonpartner sexual violence*. Geneva: World Health Organization.

Xavier, J. (2000). *Transgender Needs Assessment Survey final report for phase two*. Washington DC: Administration for HIV/AIDS of the District of Columbia.

Yavorsky, J. E., & Sayer, L. (2013). "Doing fear" The influence of hetero-femininity on (trans)women's fears of victimization. *The Sociological Quarterly*, *54*(4), 511–533.

4

TRANSGENDER MEN AND PREGNANCY

Rosie Charter, Jane M. Ussher, Janette Perz and Kerry H. Robinson

Introduction

Transgender (trans) men are commonly born with the reproductive anatomy that allows them to become pregnant and give birth, and many wish to do so (Besse, Lampe, & Mann, 2020; Obedin-Maliver & Makadon, 2016). With recent cultural shifts in community and legal attitudes around the trans community, the openness of trans men desiring parenthood and becoming parents through gestational pregnancy may be more a reality now than ever before (Tornello & Bos, 2017). Whilst there is a growing body of research around trans parenting (Charter, Ussher, Perz, & Robinson, 2022; Riggs, 2013, 2020; Walks, 2015), there is still little known about the experiences of Australian trans men negotiating parenthood and gestational pregnancy, the focus of this chapter. Data used throughout is taken from a study conducted by Charter, Ussher, Perz and Robinson (2018). Twenty-five trans men, aged 25 to 46 years old, who had experienced gestational pregnancy shared their experiences through an online survey and one-on-one interviews.

Pregnancy and Masculinity

Arguably, there is no human experience more gendered than pregnancy. Dominant reproductive discourses are founded on that irrevocability; pregnancy is gender done 'correctly', the natural progression of femininity, and its accomplishment is socially and institutionally reinforced and rewarded (Cameron, 1998; Ryan, 2013; West & Zimmerman, 1987). Even though we have witnessed the development of new technologies that challenge and expand our understanding of human reproduction, it still seems to firmly privilege heterocisnormativity. Hegemonic cultural representations of pregnancy as unique to cisgender women reinforce this. Thus, pregnancy ceases to be a 'condition' and becomes an 'identity' (Radi, 2020). Certain

DOI: 10.4324/9781003138310-4

reproducers are privileged as legitimate and others as illegitimate (Weissman, 2017). Pearce and White write: "There exists a tendency to both exceptionalize and render invisible trans reproduction, through sensationalized coverage of 'pregnant men'" (2019, p. 765). Whilst positioned as an oddity many trans men retain their reproductive organs and pursue gestational pregnancy (Epstein, 2016; Hoffkling, Obedin-Maliver, & Sevelius, 2017; Obedin-Maliver & Makadon, 2016; Riggs, Pfeffer, Pearce, Hines, & White, 2021). In Australia, official health records indicate 246 men gave birth between 2013 and 2020 (Medicare, 2020). However, given not all trans men are legally recognized by their gender marker, or may not at the time of giving birth, the actual number may be higher. Trans pregnancy essentially is, as Dietz (2021) states, "unexceptional" (p.191), people who have both the capacity and wish to become pregnant, can and will. However, the response from many healthcare providers (HCPs), institutions, and the broader community transforms male pregnancy into a social and medical 'emergency', deeply troubling the sanctity of hegemonic femininity and repronormativity (Dietz, 2021; Weissman, 2017).

There are numerous systemic barriers designed to regulate who is, and who is not, permitted to become a parent (Dietz, 2021). There are many countries which require trans people to undergo complete sterilization in order to attain legal recognition of their gender marker (Honkasalo, 2018; Riggs, Pfeffer, Pearce, Hines, & White, 2020). These types of policies have been referred to as 'passive eugenics', legislating the relinquishing of reproductive rights in order to prove trans authenticity (Bowman, 1996; Lowik, 2018; Radi, 2020); another example of systemic reinforcement that parenthood and trans identities should be antithetical, "a single narrative enacted into law that establishes and reifies a dominant norm" (Lowik, 2018, p. 427).

For trans men who are living in countries where they *can* exercise their reproductive rights, this freedom is still not necessarily guaranteed. As Dietz writes: "systematic barriers are quotidian aspects of reproductive institutions: of the doctors, hospitals, insurance policies, ethicists, and other actors that together produce the conditions of possibility for contemporary western reproduction" (2021, p. 190). With equitable treatment, trans men who have retained their reproductive organs have similar pregnancy outcomes to cisgender women (Leung, Sakkas, Pang, Thornton, & Resetkova, 2019). Whilst every pregnant person has individual clinical considerations, a shared issue for some trans men relates to the use of hormonal treatment for gender affirmation. For those who do use it, hormonal therapy, such as testosterone, will have to cease for the duration of the pregnancy. Whilst it is possible to become pregnant when taking testosterone, it is highly teratogenic to a foetus and must be discontinued if a viable pregnancy is to continue (Hembree et al., 2017). Most trans men cease taking hormones in preparation for pregnancy (Hoffkling et al., 2017). However, this can have significant implications for mental health as, for many, hormones can be a vital component of a healthcare plan and ceasing their use can exacerbate gender dysphoria and associated mental health issues (Ellis, Wojnar, & Pettinato, 2015). If medical interventions are able to be bypassed, by conceiving using known donor sperm and at-home insemination, or through intercourse, positive and straight forward experiences are generally reported (Riggs et al., 2020). However, for the many trans men who need to access medically assisted reproduction (AR), experiences are often challenging (James-Abra et al., 2015; Riggs et al., 2020).

Ethical debates regarding medical AR and who has "the right to reproduce" (De Wert et al., 2014, p. 1859) have long upheld heterocisnormative regulation of who can and cannot become a parent, accompanied by paternalistic discourses around "the best interests of the child" (Ethics Committee of the American Society for Reproductive Medicine, 2015; Hembree et al., 2017). Australian heterosexual couples have been accessing AR since 1980 (Baird, 2012; Leeton, 2004), whereas federal legislation ostensibly enshrining trans people's medical right to equal treatment was not enacted until 2013 (Australian Human Rights Commission, 2013). However, as with many aspects of trans healthcare, 'permission' to access a service does not mean that service will be granted, nor that it will be of an equitable standard. Trans people are still routinely subjected to discrimination and suboptimum care when trying to access AR (James-Abra et al., 2015; Riggs et al., 2020). In these environments, heterocisnormativity is the default, in which all systems are grounded (Light, Obedin-Maliver, Sevelius, & Kerns, 2014). Trans identities, bodies, and relationships are deeply troubling to reproductive *and* medical hegemony. As such, trans men engaging these institutions are often subjected to significant problematizing of their care by HCPs and ancillary staff, gatekeeping, and potentially having to engage multiple facilities to find one who will both grant, and then fulfil, treatment (Hoffkling et al., 2017; Moseson et al., 2021; Nixon, 2013). Thus, Riggs et al. (2020) argue that trans men must ultimately weigh "suboptimal treatment against the desire for conception" (p.14).

An additional barrier concerning trans men and gestational parenthood exists in the dialectical tension between masculinity and fecundity. Research by Riggs (2013) details the complex negotiations pregnant trans men must engage in to navigate tensions between their masculine self and the gendered expectations from inhabiting a fecund and pregnant body. Trans men may need to reconcile, or reach a personal compromise, between heterocisnormative assumptions around pregnant bodies and their own experiences of gendered embodiment. Whilst not universal, many trans men experience significant gender dysphoria throughout pregnancy, birth, and well into the postnatal period (Riggs, 2020). Ongoing gendered assumptions can be highly challenging to someone already experiencing dysphoria, especially in a medical setting. As such, gender affirming obstetric care has significant benefits in alleviating pregnancy-related dysphoria and distress (Besse et al., 2020; Hahn, Sheran, Weber, Cohan, & Obedin-Maliver, 2019; Jarin, 2019). As Obedin-Maliver and Makadon (2016) assert: whilst clinical care for trans men is in the realm of routine obstetrics, culturally competent medical and mental health care is vital for the wellbeing of parent and child.

To date, there is a need for research exploring Australian trans men's desire for parenthood, and the ways in which they negotiate, construct, and experience gestational pregnancy. This research is needed in order to allow HCPs to offer an informed dialogue around fertility preservation, conception, and prenatal support, and to support trans men's wellbeing during their pregnancy and into the postnatal period. A greater understanding may also help expand the inclusivity and visibility of trans people in reproductive and broader health literature.

The data from this chapter is taken from is part of a larger project titled "The Constructions and Experiences of Parenthood amongst Transgender Australians". This larger study was open to any transgender person in Australia who was also a parent. A mixed-methods research design using online survey data and one-on-one interviews was used to explore the parenting experiences of 66 trans individuals. This chapter examines the experiences of a subset of that broader study population: 25 trans men who had experienced a gestational pregnancy. These participants were aged 24–46 years old (*M* 35.6, *SD* 6.66), and had gestational children ranging in age from three years to 12 years old. Twenty-four participants had one gestational pregnancy, and one participant had experienced two gestational pregnancies. The majority of participants also parented other children, whom they had not carried gestationally.

Trans men's perspectives on becoming a parent

"Growing up female": The assumption of motherhood

In contemporary western society, the successful expression of womanhood is grounded in fecundity, with motherhood positioned as central to female identity, and described as a motherhood mandate (Clisby & Holdsworth, 2016; Lowe, 2016; Nash, 2012). The majority of participants we spoke to reported that the expectation of future motherhood was impressed upon them from an early age. As these participants were growing up questioning or feeling at odds with their assigned female gender identity, this mandate was reported to be particularly troubling:

> They always seemed to put it (motherhood) right at the forefront of my future, right from the get go. Be good girl, you grow up, have kids, be a mum. Everything else felt very … secondary to that …. (For me) those were extremely troublesome ideas at the time. I just really shut off.
>
> *(Tony, age 34)*

Many participants echoed this account and reported that "when you're growing up female" motherhood is positioned as "nonnegotiable" or "assumed" and that to diverge or question that narrative, as Stevie (46) notes, "makes you feel even less normal than you already do". This "assumption of fecundity" was reported to be "deeply isolating" and, for many, exacerbated struggles with gender identity; as Regan (37) said, "I just felt so shut off … from the future. I couldn't imagine that future version of myself (as a mother), or any version, and it made me feel quite alone and angry, actually".

Many participant accounts detailed isolating messages from the people close to them, which reinforced this sense of isolation or 'estrangement':

> When I was growing up, people always talked about becoming a mum, my family, their friends talked about it … You'd see women on TV being pregnant and having babies. I think I pretended to feel the same but truthfully I felt completely estranged by the idea … I could in no way picture myself doing the same.
>
> *(Roy, 24)*

Others described these early notions of becoming a parent, or specifically a mother, as "alien" or "unimaginable", as Stevie (46) said, the "idea of becoming, and being, a mother was completely foreign to me". Tommy (27) shared this account from when he was 11 years old:

> [An employee of my parents] reached out and, kind of, gently squeezed my [breast]. It wasn't sexual at all. She made this comment about how it would breastfeed a baby one day, like it was already marked out just for that … it made me feel so mixed up and horrible about my body.

Experiences of a schism between how one feels and how one is perceived are not uncommon in accounts of young trans people (McGuire, Doty, Catalpa, & Ola, 2016). However, what can make these experiences so acutely alienating is that they are often driven by those closest to us, thus depriving young trans people of a support system (Johnson & Amella, 2014; McConnell, Birkett, & Mustanski, 2016).

In the majority of accounts, participants drew on experiences across their childhood, adolescence, and into young adulthood, when they had little control over how their gender was constructed and categorized by those around them. At this time, they were particularly vulnerable to dominant cultural narratives that associated femininity with fecundity. Many participants chose to deal with perceived "maternal pressures" when they were younger by actively resisting and rejecting the motherhood mandate, as Marco (27) states: "For a long time I think I overcompensated by being very anti-children and, sort of, belittling motherhood as weak". Colin (46) said: "I was very much against becoming a mother, actually, before I came out … I thought at the time it was about keeping my independence". Other participants described parenthood variously as "a feminist issue" and "a form of control" over parents, or specifically mothers, that they wanted to resist. When asked what about parenthood was initially unappealing to him, Stefan (41) gave the following account:

> In retrospect, I think it was part of my dismissal of all things, sort of, feminine about myself and (motherhood) seemed a huge part of that female character … It just seemed easier to put it aside. I threw myself into work and tried to forget about it.

Over time, however, participants began to reconcile notions of parenthood with their bourgeoning understanding of their gender identity and how they fit in their individual world.

Orientating toward fatherhood: "Parenting on my own terms"

Previous researchers have noted that when dominant narratives are exclusionary, people will seek meaning through the creation of alternative narratives, which are crucial in allowing them to make sense of their experiences (Dryden, Ussher, & Perz, 2014; McKenzie-Mohr & Lafrance, 2011). For many participants, the desire to become a parent was kindled when they 'came out' as trans or started to pursue GA. This shift of identity from "potential mother" to "potential father" was a powerful experience, giving many "a way to imagine parenting" (Tommy, 27). As Tommy (27) says: "Once I came to terms with being trans, the idea of being a parent, and a father, began to really excite me". Others had similar experiences of "beginning to orientate toward fatherhood" post 'coming out', describing experiences such as "picturing myself as a father made it all seem suddenly very possible and exciting" (Stefan, 41) and "realizing that I could negotiate parenting on my own terms, as a dad, was really liberating" (Regan, 37). Noel (36) shared this account:

> It was right after I started on T (testosterone) … I just felt so well, I was finally living authentically and I could have a family. That, that part of my life didn't have to be, sort of, denied. I was always meant to be a father.

These accounts demonstrate the transformative power of 'coming out' and pursuing GA, wherein participants renegotiated parenthood identities to bring them into alignment with their experiences of masculine gender. This shifting of identities facilitated the ability to challenge both personal and societal assumptions around their capabilities of parenthood. In keeping with Berkowitz's (2007) work on procreative consciousness, as trans men create and negotiate 'new' narratives around parenthood and gain acknowledgement of their fatherhood identities, the potential for other trans men to imagine themselves as parents and fathers also grows significantly.

Pursuing pregnancy

Whilst becoming a parent does not always necessitate carrying a child and giving birth oneself, each of the trans men in our study made a deliberate and informed decision to pursue a pregnancy. However, in doing so, they had to engage in a complex negotiation with their masculine identity, the traditional association of pregnancy with femininity, and the material reality of the medical and biological aspects of pregnancy post-GA.

A functional sacrifice

The participants in our study chose to pursue pregnancy for a variety of reasons. Some participants had cisgender female partners whose fertility was affected by medical issues, as Sam (32) describes:

> [My partner's] endometriosis was really severe … when we started talking about a family I just knew it wasn't going to be possible for her [to get pregnant] so I decided that I'd do it. It wasn't an altogether happy decision but I knew it was the right one for us and I feel, actually, very grateful that I could do that for us.

For other participants, being able to have a child that was biologically related to them was positioned as important and valuable: "It just seemed like a huge privilege to be able to have a child that shared my DNA" (Justin, 30). Equally, Bill (31) commented:

> We'd had some close friends who'd really struggled with not being genetically related to their kids … it really made an impression on me and (my partner) … so we decided we'd take turns having a baby.

Some participants reported that they wanted to have a child before pursuing GA "took them too far" whereas others expressed the desire to "get something positive out of a body that had always felt like a curse". In these accounts, pregnancy was positioned as a "functional sacrifice", which Epstein (2016) describes as "something to endure in service of a long-term pragmatic goal" (p. 751).

"The struggle": living without T

For many of the trans men in our study, going on testosterone represented their first line of treatment after 'coming out' as trans, and was experienced as a significant validation of their masculine gender identity. However, for participants wanting to conceive, tapering off their dosage of testosterone was the first step and, for many, this was a significantly challenging experience, as Zak (29) states:

> It was really gradual at first. Then I noticed my body started to change, like my fat started to kind of shift, redistribute, around my body … my hips started coming back … my empty boobs started to really ache and then I got my period. Even though I knew it was going to happen that was still a huge shock. I had a real moment then. Like, I questioned whether I could go through with everything.

Other participants echoed these sentiments, stating that "going off T was extremely stressful", and that it "felt like my lifeline was being taken away". Trent (36) stated: "It really triggered old feelings I had about myself, I kept flashing back to being 16 again, wondering what the hell was wrong with me". Other participants described feeling distressed as a result of perceived changes such as "losing my muscle", accompanied by "lack of energy", "intense mood swings", "feeling depressed", and "flat". These are common experiences when withdrawing from testosterone (Davis & Colton Meier, 2014), but are also "symptoms" associated with the "monstrous feminine" changes across the reproductive life cycle, and signifiers of a fecund body out of control (Ussher, 2006). Some participants "fell pregnant straight away", whilst others, such as Jonnie (28) took longer, having to live with dissonance at inhabiting a feminine body not feeling "normal":

> We didn't get pregnant for almost a year, so my body had reverted back to much of its former self. I still had a little fluff on the face but everything else was really soft and round. I hated it so much. I didn't always 'pass' anymore, which was really demoralizing … Ultimately, getting pregnant was a huge relief because then I had a timeline to when I could get back to normal [laughs].

The decision to go off testosterone can be a physically and emotionally complicated one. As mental health-related quality of life, depression, and anxiety are significantly improved in trans men who receive testosterone, withdrawing from this medication could have significant implications for wellbeing (Davis & Colton Meier, 2014; Gómez-Gil et al., 2012; Newfield, Hart, Dibble, & Kohler, 2006). Additionally, the loss of the masculinizing effect of testosterone, combined with the visual presentation of a pregnancy, can have a deleterious impact on a trans man's ability to 'pass.' This can be highly distressing (Light et al., 2014; Newfield et al., 2006) and for many can compound experiences of isolation.

Accessing reproductive assistance

It has been well established that trans men face significant difficulties when accessing care and support for their reproductive health and wellbeing, and assisted fertility is no exception (Coleman et al., 2012; Pitts, Couch, Mulcare, Croy, & Mitchell, 2009; Reisner, Perkovich, & Mimiaga, 2010). As 18 of the 25 participants in this study were partnered with cisgender women at the time of conceiving children, they would not be able to conceive their children without accessing some form of external support, such as pursuing formal or informal assisted fertility, including the acquisition and insemination of donor sperm, and, in some cases, in vitro fertilization.

For many participants, accessing sperm was the first step toward conceiving their child. This generally involved two options. Firstly, using a known donor, such as a friend or colleague and generally doing a 'DIY' insemination in an informal setting such as a home. The alternative, using an unknown donor, relies on accessing a fertility clinic and having insemination done at a facility by a medical professional. The majority of participants in our study used informal channels to acquire and use sperm, as Colin (46) explains: "For us, using a (known donor) was so much easier 'cause we could just do everything at home … We were extremely lucky and it worked on the second go". Mickie (33) explains further:

> Once we decided to use a known donor … it was really just a matter of approaching them and discussing what we were proposing. It's tricky because the legal side of it was a bit of grey area at the time and we really just had to keep it to ourselves and hope for the best, to be honest … We were really lucky that [the donor] was keen and shared our feelings about what his relationship would be with [our child].

These accounts were echoed by other participants, who found "the negotiation process much easier" with a known donor, and DIY insemination "much easier", "more personal", and "less confronting" than accessing formal facilities. As Trent (36) describes: "We did (the insemination) at home … and, you know, rather than being weird or impersonal it was actually all very special". However, experiences of assisted fertility were very different for those participants who chose to use formal fertility services. Many described it as a "nightmare process" that none were able to see through to completion. We were rejected from multiple clinics due to "reasons unknown". "We had a range of appointments and each time the discussion centred almost completely on my gender identity … everyone just seemed so uncomfortable seeing us" (Justin, 30). Other participants echoed this account, describing "embarrassing" and "awkward" appointments followed by "cancelling our follow-ups". Trent (36) stated: "The doctor we saw was so awkward with us, kept misgendering me and repeatedly asked why my (cisgender) partner wasn't the one to have the baby". For these participants, dealing with negative experiences with fertility service providers was "the first in many pregnancy-related rejections and disappointments" (Noel, 36).

Whilst trans people are protected legally in Australia from discrimination by HCPs (New South Wales Government, 1977), these protections are not necessarily born out in their actual experiences. No participant in this study who attempted to access a fertility clinic was actually granted treatment. This type of rejection and discrimination is reported to be pervasive in the trans community, and has a very significant impact on mental health and wellbeing (Rood et al., 2016). As such, like many in the broader LGBTQI community, trans men turn to informal networks and methods, indicated in the above accounts of using known donors and at-home insemination, to assist them in achieving their goal to conceive.

The pregnant man

Inhabiting the pregnant body

For many participants, pregnancy-related physical changes brought with them an unexpected psychological and emotional toll. Bill (31) explains:

The happiness at getting that [positive result] was pretty quickly replaced with a sense of real dread ... the early hormones made me feel really sick and shaky and I think the enormity of what I was doing really started to sink in and I got scared.

For others, the pregnant body was experienced as "frightening", "distressing", and "extremely difficult to handle". Tommy (27) noted "the changes (to my body) really disgusted me. It was a very stressful time". Changes such as "weight gain", "breast growth", "breast tenderness", as well as looking both "more feminine" and "less masculine" were the most commonly cited causes for distress. For these participants, pregnancy was an overwhelming experience that compounded and complicated what Regan termed the experience of a "complete dysphoria of the body":

I felt completely in the wrong body, my flesh, the roundness and bulges, the way it felt and looked, really frightened me, so foreign, like the more pregnant I got the more alien my skin felt. It terrified me. It wasn't the femaleness of it, it was the intense changes, the physical changes.

(Regan, 37)

Many participants reported dealing with these acute experiences of pregnancy-related dysphoria by "distancing", "detaching", and "disassociating" themselves from their pregnant bodies. As Wyn (42) says: "In order to cope, I had to detach ... I ended up so detached from my (pregnant) body that I sometimes needed to be reminded that I was pregnant". Tommy (27) echoed this account, stating that: "As (the pregnancy) kept progressing I got more and more anxious ... detaching kind of helped me cope in the short term ... I gave myself permission to do whatever I needed to just get through".

Detaching, as a coping strategy, is not uncommon when dealing with acute stressors and is viewed as an adaptive coping method (Elklit, 1996; Roger, Jarvis, & Najarian, 1993). Creating distance between oneself and the stressor can bring with it the cognitive space needed to cope and get through challenging experiences (Elklit, 1996).

Chest distress

The visual presence of 'breasts' is a key signifier of adult femininity (Goin & Goin, 1981; Spencer, 1996). Many trans men refer to this area of their body as their 'chest', whilst some refer to it as their 'breasts', or use the terms interchangeably depending on factors, such as where they may be in their pursuit of GA (Davis & Colton Meier, 2014; MacDonald et al., 2016). As such, for the trans men in our study, changes to the chest were experienced as the most challenging pregnancy-related physical change. As Regan (37) describes: "it was really stressful feeling my breasts grow so much, it made me feel sick". Stefan (41) concurs "they [chest] got huge and it was extremely stressful, I didn't like to look at them, or touch them". Other participants stated that they "hated looking at" themselves due to chest changes.

Strategies normally used to conceal the chest, such as binding (MacDonald et al., 2016) were not as effective during pregnancy, with many participants unable to bind at all. This was described as "a real struggle", "very difficult", "challenging", and "extremely uncomfortable". As Jason (26) explains: "not being able to bind was a nightmare. My chest was getting so big it was totally impossible to cover … people started misgendering me, a lot, which hurt". For many, being unable to bind led to the decision to completely isolate themselves, and "hide out", due to "fear of being outed", or experiencing "shame" or "self-consciousness". As Noel (36) says:

> [Towards the end of pregnancy] I just stopped leaving the house completely … I felt really unsafe and anxious when I was out and it just wasn't worth it, in the end … I couldn't bind and I felt so uncomfortable in my body. I hated being seen. I felt like everyone was staring.

For some, this period of isolation was not just confined to pregnancy but continued well into the postnatal period:

> [My chest] was huge and leaky after I had [my child] … It was so horrible and totally stressed me out … I couldn't bind because it was way too painful … it was also right in the middle of summer and it was so hot. I couldn't cover up, I couldn't bind. I ended up just staying home for months, which sounds simple but it was super isolating.
>
> *(Sam, 32)*

Post-birth chestfeeding was also a significant issue for participants. For many, it was described as "trigger(ing) intense dysphoria" and was "deeply distressing". As Bailey (25) says: "breastfeeding, for me, represented the absolute pinnacle of my dysphoria, unbelievably bad". Support from partners was integral during this time, with many participants stating that it "saved" them: "I was so relieved when my partner supported me to not chestfeed, I really don't think I could've coped with that" (Clarence, 43).

Given their overwhelming association with fecundity and femininity, "breasts" are considered by some to be the physical attribute most in conflict with a male gender identity (Davis & Colton Meier, 2014; Spencer, 1996). As illustrated by participant accounts, changes to this area of the body can have far-reaching and significant implications for the wellbeing of pregnant trans men, making this period of their lives much more difficult.

The isolation of exclusion: "Am I the only one?"

People who deviate from normative expectations of gender disrupt the societal assumption that gender expression strictly adheres to one's assigned biological sex (Ryan, 2013). To diverge from this assumption can open oneself up to acute discrimination and social exclusion. It could be argued that the pregnant man transgresses these normative expectations of gender more than any other (Karaian, 2013). As such, for the men in our study, pregnancy brought with it much isolation and exclusion. As one participant stated, "For all the joy pregnancy should have brought, there were a huge amount of constraints put on me, and it was very, very isolating" (Jason, 26). Some participants expressed that they were "locked out of being able to really experience pregnancy", or as Colin (46) explains:

> I can't express how lonely it was to go through a whole pregnancy in hiding. I couldn't be 'out' as a pregnant person and it was really hard. Like, yes my friends and family knew but to the rest of the world I had to hide it to protect my own safety and my mental health from strangers. The loneliness was profound.

Others concurred that social exclusion stemming from "not confirming to what a pregnant person is supposed to look like" fuelled isolation and loneliness:

> I just felt so lonely, like "am I the only one?". There was no one at the doctors or the clinic or in the pregnancy books or anywhere like me. I felt like a complete anomaly.
>
> *(Noel, 36)*

Although there have been no studies on perinatal depression in trans men, experiences of isolation and loneliness during pregnancy have been linked to perinatal depression in cisgender women (Bonari et al., 2004; Leung & Kaplan, 2009), and thus our participants could also be vulnerable to developing this condition. Within the context of this isolation and loneliness existed also the "lack of representation" of what a male pregnancy might look like. Zak (29) gave this account:

> Not seeing yourself [represented] anywhere is so hard. I felt like I was really excluded from the whole thing [of pregnancy] and I didn't get any enjoyment from it. Reading the books, or looking on the internet for pregnancy advice was so depressing. It felt like it was just a constant barrage of information confirming how wrong I was.

These feelings were contextualized by others, commenting on the "complete lack of resources", "invisibility of trans men" in pregnancy literature, and the "complete lack of specialized support" for pregnant trans men. Invisibility and marginalization due to gender identity is common in health research, and trans men, amongst others in the broader LGBTQI community, have been excluded from mainstream health-promotion research, policy, and practice (Mulé et al., 2009).

Discussion

For the trans men in our study, early experiences of pressure to become a parent through fulfilling the "motherhood mandate" were both confronting and alienating, leading to feelings of exclusion from dominant parenting narratives. Heterocisnormativity creates an expectation of motherhood for all those who are identified as 'woman' (Obedin-Maliver & Makadon, 2016; Page & Peacock, 2013), with 'woman' and 'mother' being treated as synonymous. The fecund body has thus "been socially gendered as unquestioningly feminine because of its association with female-bodied people" (Ryan, 2013, p. 119). In the majority of accounts of negotiating desire for parenthood, or of resisting the motherhood mandate, participants drew on experiences across their childhood, adolescence, and into young adulthood, when they had little control over how their gender was constructed and categorized by those around them. At this time, they were particularly vulnerable to dominant cultural narratives that associated femininity with fecundity. However, upon 'coming out' and commencing GA, participants were able to negotiate and construct their own parenting identity. These findings illustrate the significance that 'coming out' and pursuing GA can have in bringing a sense of congruence to trans men's lives (Fein, Salgado, Alvarez, & Estes, 2017), which in turn enables them to move forward in ways important to them, such as pursuing a pregnancy.

Trans men who make the decision to become parents must do so whilst navigating in a world designed to exclude. Healthcare systems are not generally supportive of trans bodies and identities (Conron, Scott, Stowell, & Landers, 2012; Pitts et al., 2009) and it is telling that none of the men in our study were successfully treated at any fertility clinic that they attended, even though their right to treatment is, technically, protected in Australia (Anti-Discrimination Board of New South Wales, 2011; Easten, 2002; New South Wales Government, 1977). The majority of the participants in our study thus relied on informal methods to conceive their children. However, this leaves them 'locked out' of formalized treatments and support networks. Not everyone is comfortable with, or able to find, a known donor, nor to use at-home insemination successfully. Thus, our research illustrates that some trans men are experiencing exclusion from pursuing gestational pregnancies through structural exclusion and discriminatory practices. Every staff member of these organizations, from those administrators on the front desk, to the nurses, pathologists, and doctors who treat patients, needs to be educated on how to negotiate an inclusive and supportive provision of their service to those in the community.

For many trans men, hormone therapy is experienced as essential to combating gender dysphoria and bringing one's gender into alignment (Nelson, 2016). The results from our study indicate that ceasing hormone therapy during the preconception period can trigger distressing dysphoric episodes and, as evidenced in the above accounts, can set a troubling pattern for the subsequent pregnancy. Pregnancy-related dysphoria was a huge issue for participants and one that is currently an unknown quantity for many HCPs (MacDonald et al., 2016; Obedin-Maliver & Makadon, 2016; Veale, Watson, Adjei, & Saewyc, 2016). The preconception, prenatal, and perinatal periods pose many challenges for trans men, and they must navigate these experiences without, what is for many, a key treatment, testosterone. As such, HCPs and trans men alike need to develop a better understanding of how to manage gender dysphoria when hormonal therapies are not an option during the pre- and perinatal periods.

The 'breasts' project has many cues associated with femininity and for pregnant trans men the growing pregnant chest is experienced as extremely troubling. The majority of the trans men in our study had not undergone subcutaneous mastectomy, or top surgery, and still retained their original chest tissue during their pregnancies. As such, their growing chest triggered intense dysphoria. This had a number of implications, such as poor parental mental health, but also impacted on whether the participant's chest fed their babies. Whilst one study found trans men are comfortable chest feeding (MacDonald et al., 2016), the majority of men in our study found it too confronting and either chose not to, or only chest fed for a matter of weeks. The decision of how to feed one's baby is a very personal one for all new parents, but for trans men this choice must be balanced between the well-established health benefits of chest feeding and the challenges that such a practice might sustain (Obedin-Maliver & Makadon, 2016). Specialized resources need to be developed to support trans men in relation to pregnancy-related chest changes and lactation specialists and community nurses need to be trained in supporting trans men and their babies in the postnatal period.

Ellis et al. (2015) wrote, of their study into the conception, pregnancy, and birth experiences of gender variant parents: "loneliness was the overarching theme that permeated all participants' experiences, social interactions, and emotional responses through every stage of achieving gestational parenthood" (p. 63). This statement could be made from our own findings as experiences of profound isolation and loneliness overarched our own participants' accounts. A large body of research illustrates the connection between these experiences and an increased risk for postnatal depression, which could have serious implications for parental health and the health of their babies, both in the immediate postnatal period and into the future (Bonari et al., 2004; Wisner, 2009). Additionally, as baseline depression, self-harm, and suicide rates are higher amongst trans individuals than the broader population, particular attention to postnatal depression is certainly warranted (Obedin-Maliver & Makadon, 2016). However, there is currently negligible research on trans men's experiences of peri- and postnatal depression. To fully explore this area and aid in the development of resources that are more trans inclusive, more research is warranted.

This research demonstrates that trans men are having babies and are doing so without the formal support and resources that they not only need but have a right to. This leaves many feeling isolated, excluded, and vulnerable during a time when support is most required. Whilst there may be specialized HCPs who are knowledgeable about trans men's reproductive and obstetric health, it is unlikely that there are enough to support this population. Additionally, given the prevalence of discrimination experienced by trans people within the healthcare system (Grant et al., 2011; Mulé et al., 2009; Scheim, Zong, Giblon, & Bauer, 2017), work needs to be done by HCPs and others in the community to make reproductive health more inclusive of trans bodies and identities. Education of HCPs with regard to transgender issues and reproductive health is also necessary in order to counteract the lack of knowledge in this area and to stem the discrimination that prevails. Further, the current study illuminated an area of research that requires urgent attention, and that is the experiences of transgender men when accessing assisted fertility services. Future enquiries must also include trans men who have not been able to conceive, which may be associated with access to services, in order to provide a more inclusive picture of trans men's experiences of their fertility and pregnancy. Additionally, it may provide further insight into ways in which the provision of fertility services and information can be improved for trans men, and the broader trans community, who remain largely underrepresented in reproductive health research.

For the pregnant trans man, the materiality of the pregnant body is at odds with their identities as men and the subject position 'father'. Whilst GA can bring one's gender and embodied experience into alignment, the requirements of pursuing pregnancy serve to disrupt this alignment at a vulnerable time for any prospective parent. It is telling, perhaps that most of the participants in our study are yet to pursue a second pregnancy. This research also troubles static notions of 'fatherhood' and 'motherhood', suggesting that subject positions can be negotiated by individuals, even if this is at odds with their embodied experience, or how their body is viewed by others. The findings of this study are important insofar as they provide insight into how trans men experience and construct gestational parenthood and pregnancy. We hope that the body of research into trans men's experiences of pregnancy and parenthood can continue to be explored, and that appropriate services and resources for this population can be developed and delivered.

References

Anti-Discrimination Board of New South Wales. (2011). *Transgender Discrimination Factsheet*. Retrieved from www.antidiscrimination.justice.nsw.gov.au/Documents/Transgender-discrimination-factsheet-Jul2015.pdf

Australian Human Rights Commission. (2013). Sexual orientation, gender identity & intersex status discrimination: Information sheet. Retrieved from https://humanrights.gov.au/our-work/lgbti/projects/new-protection

Baird, B. (2012). An Australian history of lesbian mothers: Two points of emergence. *Women's History Review, 21*(5), 849–865.

Berkowitz, D. (2007). A sociohistorical analysis of gay men's procreative consciousness. *Journal of GLBT Family Studies, 3*(2–3), 157–190.

Besse, M., Lampe, N. M., & Mann, E. S. (2020). Experiences with achieving pregnancy and giving birth among transgender men: A narrative literature review. *The Yale journal of Biology & Medicine, 93*(4), 517–528.

Bonari, L., Pinto, N., Ahn, E., Einarson, A., Steiner, M., & Koren, G. (2004). Perinatal risks of untreated depression during pregnancy. *The Canadian Journal of Psychiatry, 49*(11), 726–735.

Bowman, J. E. (1996). The road to eugenics. *University of Chicago Law School Roundtable, 3*, 491.

Cameron, D. (1998). Performing gender identity. In J. Coates (Ed.), *Language and gender: A reader*. Oxford: Blackwell.

Charter, R., Ussher, J. M., Perz, J., & Robinson, K. (2018). The transgender parent: Experiences and constructions of pregnancy and parenthood for transgender men in Australia. *International Journal of Transgenderism, 19*(1), 64–77.

Charter, R., Ussher, J. M., Perz, J., & Robinson, K. H. (2022). Negotiating mental health amongst transgender parents in Australia. *International Journal of Transgender Health, 23*(3), 308–320.

Clisby, S., & Holdsworth, J. (2016). *Gendering women: Identity and mental wellbeing through the lifecourse.* Bristol, UK: Policy Press.

Coleman, E., Bockting, W., Botzer, M., Cohen-Kettenis, P., DeCuypere, G., Feldman, J., … Zucker, K. (2012). Standards of care for the health of transsexual, transgender, and gender-nonconforming people, version 7. *International Journal of Transgenderism, 13*(4), 165–232.

Conron, K. J., Scott, G., Stowell, G. S., & Landers, S. (2012). Transgender health in Massachusetts: Results from a household probability sample of adults. *American Journal of Public Health, 102*(1), 118–122.

Davis, S. A., & Colton Meier, S. (2014). Effects of testosterone treatment and chest reconstruction surgery on mental health and sexuality in female-to-male transgender people. *International Journal of Sexual Health, 26*(2), 113–128.

De Wert, G., Dondorp, W., Shenfield, F., Barri, P., Devroey, P., Diedrich, K., … Pennings, G. (2014). ESHRE Task Force on Ethics and Law 23: Medically assisted reproduction in singles, lesbian and gay couples, and transsexual people†. *Human Reproduction, 29*(9), 1859–1865.

Dietz, E. (2021). Normal parents: Trans pregnancy and the production of reproducers. *International Journal of Transgender Health, 22*(1–2), 191–202.

Dryden, A., Ussher, J. M., & Perz, J. (2014). Young women's construction of their post-cancer fertility. *Psychology & Health, 29*(11), 1341–1360.

Easten, R. (2002). Protecting transgender rights under Queensland's Discrimination Law Amendment Act 2002 [Press release].

Elklit, A. (1996). Coping styles questionnaire: A contribution to the validation of a scale for measuring coping strategies. *Personality and Individual Differences, 21*(5), 809–812.

Ellis, S. A., Wojnar, D. M., & Pettinato, M. (2015). Conception, pregnancy, and birth experiences of male and gender variant gestational parents: It's how we could have a family. *Journal of Midwifery & Women's Health, 60*(1), 62–69.

Epstein, R. (2016). Masculinity and pregnancy. In A. E. Goldberg (Ed.), *The SAGE encyclopedia of LGBTQ studies* (pp. 750–753). Thousand Oaks, CA: Sage.

Ethics Committee of the American Society for Reproductive Medicine. (2015). Access to fertility services by transgender persons: an Ethics Committee opinion. *Fertility and Sterility, 104*(5), 1111–1115.

Fein, L. A., Salgado, C. J., Alvarez, C. V., & Estes, C. M. (2017). Transitioning transgender: Investigating the important aspects of the transition: A brief report. *International Journal of Sexual Health, 29*(1), 80–88.

Goin, M. K., & Goin, J. M. (1981). Midlife reactions to mastectomy and subsequent breast reconstruction. *Archives of General Psychiatry, 38*(2), 225–227.

Gómez-Gil, E., Zubiaurre-Elorza, L., Esteva, I., Guillamon, A., Godás, T., Cruz Almaraz, M., … Salamero, M. (2012). Hormone-treated transsexuals report less social distress, anxiety and depression. *Psychoneuroendocrinology, 37*(5), 662–670.

Grant, J. M., Mottet, L. A., Tanis, J., Harrison, J., Herman, J. L., & Keisling, M. (2011). *Injustice at every turn: A report of the national transgender discrimination survey.* Retrieved from www.thetaskforce.org/statichtml/downloads/reports/reports/ntdsfull.pdf

Hahn, M., Sheran, N., Weber, S., Cohan, D., & Obedin-Maliver, J. (2019). Providing patient-centered perinatal care for transgender men and gender-diverse individuals: A collaborative multidisciplinary team approach. *Obstetrics & Gynecology, 134*(5), 959–963.

Hembree, W. C., Cohen-Kettenis, P. T., Gooren, L., Hannema, S. E., Meyer, W. J., Murad, M. H., … T'Sjoen, G. G. (2017). Endocrine treatment of gender-dysphoric/gender-incongruent persons: An endocrine society clinical practice guideline. *The Journal of Clinical Endocrinology & Metabolism, 102*(11), 3869–3903.

Hoffkling, A., Obedin-Maliver, J., & Sevelius, J. (2017). From erasure to opportunity: A qualitative study of the experiences of transgender men around pregnancy and recommendations for providers. *BMC Pregnancy and Childbirth, 17*(2), 332.

Honkasalo, J. (2018). Unfit for parenthood? Compulsory sterilization and transgender reproductive justice in Finland. *Journal of International Women's Studies, 20*(1), 40.

James-Abra, S., Tarasoff, L. A., Green, D., Epstein, R., Anderson, S., Marvel, S., … Ross, L. E. (2015). Trans people's experiences with assisted reproduction services: a qualitative study. *Human Reproduction, 30*(6), 1365–1374.

Jarin, J. (2019). The Ob/Gyn and the transgender patient. *Current Opinion in Obstetrics and Gynecology, 31*(5), 298–302.

Johnson, M. J., & Amella, E. J. (2014). Isolation of lesbian, gay, bisexual and transgender youth: a dimensional concept analysis. *Journal of Advanced Nursing, 70*(3), 523–532.

Karaian, L. (2013). Pregnant men: Repronormativity, critical trans theory and the re(conceive)ing of sex and pregnancy in law. *Social & Legal Studies, 22*(2), 211–230.

Leeton, J. (2004). The early history of IVF in Australia and its contribution to the world (1970–1990)★. *Australian and New Zealand Journal of Obstetrics and Gynaecology, 44*(6), 495–501.

Leung, A., Sakkas, D., Pang, S., Thornton, K., & Resetkova, N. (2019). Assisted reproductive technology outcomes in female-to-male transgender patients compared with cisgender patients: A new frontier in reproductive medicine. *Fertility and Sterility, 112*(5), 858–865.

Leung, B. M., & Kaplan, B. J. (2009). Perinatal depression: Prevalence, risks, and the nutrition link—a review of the literature. *Journal of the American Dietetic Association, 109*(9), 1566–1575.

Light, A. D., Obedin-Maliver, J., Sevelius, J. M., & Kerns, J. L. (2014). Transgender men who experienced pregnancy after female-to-male gender transitioning. *Obstetrics and Gynecology, 124*(6), 1120–1127.

Lowe, P. (2016). *Reproductive health and maternal sacrifice.* London: Palgrave Macmillan.

Lowik, A. J. (2018). Reproducing eugenics, reproducing while trans: The state sterilization of trans people. *Journal of GLBT Family Studies, 14*(5), 425–445.

MacDonald, T., Noel-Weiss, J., West, D., Walks, M., Biener, M., Kibbe, A., & Myler, E. (2016). Transmasculine individuals' experiences with lactation, chestfeeding, and gender identity: A qualitative study. *BMC Pregnancy and Childbirth, 16*(106), 106.

McConnell, E. A., Birkett, M., & Mustanski, B. (2016). Families matter: Social support and mental health trajectories among lesbian, gay, bisexual, and transgender youth. *Journal of Adolescent Health, 59*(6), 674–680.

McGuire, J. K., Doty, J. L., Catalpa, J. M., & Ola, C. (2016). Body image in transgender young people: Findings from a qualitative, community based study. *Body Image, 18*, 96–107.

McKenzie-Mohr, S., & Lafrance, M. N. (2011). Telling stories without the words: "Tightrope talk" in women's accounts of coming to live well after rape or depression. *Feminism & Psychology, 21*(1), 49–73.

Medicare. (2020). Medicare Item 16519 processed from July 2013 to June 2020.

Moseson, H., Fix, L., Hastings, J., Stoeffler, A., Lunn, M. R., Flentje, A., … Obedin-Maliver, J. (2021). Pregnancy intentions and outcomes among transgender, nonbinary, and gender-expansive people assigned female or intersex at birth in the United States: Results from a national, quantitative survey. *International Journal of Transgender Health, 22*(1–2), 30–41.

Mulé, N. J., Ross, L. E., Deeprose, B., Jackson, B. E., Daley, A., Travers, A., & Moore, D. (2009). Promoting LGBT health and wellbeing through inclusive policy development. *International Journal for Equity in Health, 8*(1), 18.

Nash, M. (2012). *Making "postmodern" mothers: Pregnant embodiment, baby bumps and body image*. London: Palgrave Macmillan.

Nelson, J. L. (2016). Understanding transgender and medically assisted gender transition: Feminism as a critical resource. *AMA Journal of Ethics, 18*(11), 1132–1138.

New South Wales Government. (1977). *New South Wales Anti-Discrimination Act 1977 No 48.* www.legislation.nsw.gov.au/inforce/f38c7dc7-ba45-ee6e-d61f-9c8e3cbd52cf/1977-48. pdf

Newfield, E., Hart, S., Dibble, S., & Kohler, L. (2006). Female-to-male transgender quality of life. *Quality of Life Research, 15*(9), 1447–1457.

Nixon, L. (2013). The right to (trans) parent: a reproductive justice approach to reproductive rights, fertility, and family-building issues facing transgender people. *William & Mary Journal of Women & the Law, 20*, 73.

Obedin-Maliver, J., & Makadon, H. J. (2016). Transgender men and pregnancy. *Obstetric Medicine: The Medicine of Pregnancy, 9*, 4–8.

Page, A. D., & Peacock, J. R. (2013). Negotiating identities in a heteronormative context. *Journal of Homosexuality, 60*, 639–652.

Pearce, R., & White, F. R. (2019). Beyond the pregnant man: Representing trans pregnancy in A Deal With The Universe. *Feminist Media Studies, 19*(5), 764–767.

Pitts, M. K., Couch, M., Mulcare, H., Croy, S., & Mitchell, A. (2009). Transgender people in Australia and New Zealand: Health, well-being and access to health services. *Feminism & Psychology, 19*(4), 475–495.

Radi, B. (2020). Reproductive injustice, trans rights, and eugenics. *Sexual and Reproductive Health Matters, 28*(1), 1824318.

Reisner, S. L., Perkovich, B., & Mimiaga, M. J. (2010). A mixed methods study of the sexual health needs of New England transmen who have sex with nontransgender men. *AIDS Patient Care & STDs, 24*(8), 501–513.

Riggs, D. W. (2013). Transgender men's self-representations of bearing children post-transition. In F. Green & M. Friedman (Eds.), *Chasing rainbows: Exploring gender fluid parenting practices*. Toronto: Demeter Press.

Riggs, D. W. (2020). Transition to parenthood. In A. E. Goldberg & G. Beemyn (Eds.), *The SAGE encyclopedia of trans studies* (pp. 594–597). New York: Sage.

Riggs, D. W., Pfeffer, C. A., Pearce, R., Hines, S., & White, F. R. (2020). Men, trans/masculine, and non-binary people negotiating conception: Normative resistance and inventive pragmatism. *International Journal of Transgender Health, 22*(1–2), 6–17.

Riggs, D. W., Pfeffer, C. A., Pearce, R., Hines, S., & White, F. R. (2021). Men, trans/masculine, and non-binary people negotiating conception: Normative resistance and inventive pragmatism. *International Journal of Transgender Health, 22*(1–2), 6–17.

Roger, D., Jarvis, G., & Najarian, B. (1993). Detachment and coping: The construction and validation of a new scale for measuring coping strategies. *Personality and Individual Differences, 15*(6), 619–626.

Rood, B. A., Reisner, S. L., Surace, F. I., Puckett, J. A., Maroney, M. R., & Pantalone, D. W. (2016). Expecting rejection: Understanding the minority stress experiences of transgender and gender-nonconforming individuals. *Transgender Health, 1*, 151–164.

Ryan, M. (2013). The gender of pregnancy: Masculine lesbians talk about reproduction. *Journal of Lesbian Studies, 17*(2), 119–133.

Scheim, A. I., Zong, X., Giblon, R., & Bauer, G. R. (2017). Disparities in access to family physicians among transgender people in Ontario, Canada. *International Journal of Transgenderism, 18*(3), 343–352.

Spencer, K. W. (1996). Significance of the breast to the individual and society. *Plastic Surgery Nursing, 16*(3), 131–132.

Tornello, S. L., & Bos, H. (2017). Parenting intentions among transgender individuals. *LGBT Health, 4*(2), 115–120.

Ussher, J. M. (2006). *Managing the monstrous feminine: Regulating the reproductive body.* London: Routledge.

Veale, J., Watson, R. J., Adjei, J., & Saewyc, E. (2016). Prevalence of pregnancy involvement among Canadian transgender youth and its relation to mental health, sexual health, and gender identity. *International Journal of Transgenderism, 17*(3–4), 107–113.

Walks, M. (2015). Masculine pregnancy: Butch lesbians', trans men's & genderqueer individuals' experiences. In N. Burton (Ed.), *Natal signs: Cultural representations of pregnancy, birth, and parenting* (pp. 41–57). Toronto: Demeter Press.

Weissman, A. L. (2017). Repronormativity and the reproduction of the nation-state: The state and sexuality collide. *Journal of GLBT Family Studies, 13*(3), 277–305.

West, C., & Zimmerman, D. H. (1987). Doing gender. *Gender and Society, 1*(2), 125–151.

Wisner, K. L. (2009). Depression during pregnancy: Pregnant women need evidence-based treatment for depression. *Psychiatric Times, 26*(11), 48–50.

5

"WE NEED TO BE HEARD, RESPECTED, AND SUPPORTED"

The impact of sexual healthcare interactions and discrimination on the mental health of trans and gender diverse people

Jane M. Ussher, Bella Bushby, Chantell Sheehan, Alexandra J. Hawkey, Janette Perz, Eloise Brook and Jane Costello

Introduction

The history of trans and gender diverse (TGD)[1] healthcare has been characterised by a lack of understanding and erasure around how individuals experience their gender and sexuality. TGD people often bear the brunt of stigma and discrimination based on their gender and expression, which has significant impacts on their lives and healthcare (Balik et al., 2020). In most societies around the world, TGD people face marginalisation from multiple, often intersecting, aspects of their daily life, including legal, economic, educational, employment, housing, medical, social, and cultural forms of discrimination (James et al., 2016). At the same time, the invisibility of TGD people within population-based data collection and research continues to preclude trans health and social issues from being considered and represented within policy and resource and service allocation (Callander et al., 2019). Specifically, TGD people often face significant barriers to adequate healthcare compared to cisgender (cis) counterparts (Shires & Jaffee, 2015). This is, in part, attributable to fear, stigma, transphobia, lack of trans inclusive and specific services, and healthcare workers being under-informed of the specific needs for trans and gender diverse patients, which subsequently leads to unmet health needs and discrimination within mainstream health services (Balik, et al., 2020; Poteat, German, & Kerrigan, 2013; Ussher, Allison, Perz, Power, & The Out with Cancer Study Team, 2022a).

Trans and gender diverse people report significantly worse mental health outcomes than cis people (Hyde et al., 2014; Pitts, Smith, Mitchell, & Patel, 2006), which is a direct result of the high rates of marginalisation and discrimination they experience, described as minority stress (Carmel & Erickson-Schroth, 2016). TGD people also have lower self-reported health compared to the general Australian population, with 12.7% of TGD participants reporting their health as

DOI: 10.4324/9781003138310-5

poor (Kerr, Fisher, & Jones, 2019). When it comes to sexual health, TGD populations are recognised to be at a high risk for both sexually transmitted infections (STIs) and blood-borne viruses (BBVs) including HIV (Baral et al., 2013; Stephens, Bernstein, & Philip, 2010). According to the World Health Organization (WHO), trans women are 49 times more likely to contract HIV than the general population (World Health Organization, 2015). High rates of mental health problems have been reported in TGD people living with HIV, with medical providers identified as providing an important link to prevention, health, and support of this population (Clements-Nolle et al., 2001). However, there is consistent evidence that TGD and LGBQ (lesbian, gay, bisexual or queer) cis people postpone sexual healthcare needs and avoid obtaining healthcare services due to their fears or previous experiences of stigmatisation, with a direct result on health outcomes (Balik, et al., 2020; Shires & Jaffee, 2015). TGD people who avoid healthcare because of fear of discrimination have significantly worse outcomes than those who do not delay, or delay care for other reasons, including higher rates of depression and suicidal ideation (Seelman Colón-Diaz, LeCroix, Xavier-Brier, & Kattari, 2017).

The aim of this chapter is to examine experiences of sexual healthcare, as well as experiences of interactions with healthcare professionals, in relation to the mental health and wellbeing of TGD people. In this analysis, we draw on the findings of a recent survey of 699 TGD (binary and non-binary) people conducted in Australia, by the Positive Life NSW, The Gender Centre Inc., TGD Expert Advisory Group *2020 Trans and Gender Diverse Health and Social Needs Assessment: A Community Survey* (TGD Needs Assessment), as well as published research in this sphere.

Positive Life NSW/The Gender Centre Inc., and TGD Expert Advisory Group TGD Needs Assessment

The TGD Needs Assessment involved quantitative and qualitative survey data collected by Positive Life NSW and The Gender Centre Inc. from June 2019 to September 2019, described in detail elsewhere (Positive Life NSW, The Gender Centre Inc, & TGD Expert Advisory Group, 2020). Surveys were completed by 699 TGD participants, with ages ranging from 16 to 75 years (M 18.71, SD 13.33). Participants included 282 trans women, 150 trans men, and 267 gender diverse participants, gender groupings agreed by the Expert Advisory Group. This TGD-led research was guided by an Expert Advisory Group of nine trans and gender diverse community members, with some members openly identifying as people living with HIV. The Expert Advisory Group provided the objective and focus of the research, provided advice and guidance into the survey design, range, and type of questions ensuring appropriate language and peer representation, interpretation of results, and peer-review of the final report. The aspects of the TGD Needs Assessment reported in this chapter are experiences of sexual health screening (Positive Life NSW et al., 2020) and the association between discrimination, experiences and comfort within healthcare, gender affirmation, and self-reported mental health, and secondary analysis of the Positive Life/Gender Centre Inc/TGD Advisory Group TGD Needs Assessment data conducted as part of a Masters of ClinPsych thesis (Sheehan, 2020). Members of the Expert Advisory Group approved this chapter.

Barriers and facilitators of sexual health screening for TGD people

In response to HIV and STI policy, TGD people and TGD strategies have been largely absent from health policy approaches, clinical data, and service provision; however, this is slowly changing. International health response from UNAIDS in recent years has identified TGD people as a key population within Global AIDS Strategy 2021–26, where it is acknowledged that the risk of acquiring HIV is 13 times higher for TGD people (UNAIDS, 2015). Similarly, in 2018, the Australian Government Department of Health included TGD people as a priority population in the Eighth National HIV Strategy 2018–2022 (Australian Government Department of Health, 2018a) and within the Fourth National STI Strategy 2018–2022 (Australian Government Department of Health, 2018b). This national STI strategy identified the need for TGD people to be considered within the response to STIs and the need for improved data and research to better understand how STIs and BBVs including HIV impact TGD people.

In the TGD Needs Assessment, a minority of participants had been diagnosed or treated for STIs in their lifetime, including: Herpes (7.3%), Gonorrhoea (6.9%), Chlamydia (6.7%), Human Papillomavirus (HPV) (5.3%), Syphilis (3.3%), Hepatitis C (1.9%), and Hepatitis B (1.3%). Whilst only a minority of the survey participants, these rates are higher than those found in the general Australian population (Jasek et al., 2017). A minority (2.8%) of survey participants were living with HIV, with 82.2% HIV negative, and 13.8% had an unknown HIV status. Around two in five participants (40.1%) reported never having been tested for HIV while 59.9% reported having had at least one HIV test in their lifetime. Of those who had been tested for HIV at least once in their lifetime, only 55.9% had been tested within the past year. TGD men were more likely than all other groups to have never been tested for HIV (46.1%) (Positive Life NSW, et al., 2020). Qualitative insights revealed that some participants had low HIV risk awareness, potentially accounting for the reason why some participants had never tested for HIV. Roughly one in five (21%) of those who had never tested for HIV reported they had never had sex: "Unless I contracted HIV at birth, I have no reason to believe I could be infected"; "Never engaged in any activity that could make me HIV positive". For those who were sexually active, the most common reason provided as to why participants have never tested for HIV was lack of participation in sexual activities which participants considered risky: "I don't engage in anal play"; ""I don't fuck dudes"; "No random sexual partners"; "I've never had sex or come into any intimate contact with anyone who I knew had HIV". Several respondents commented on not engaging in injecting drug use "I don't use needles".

Most participants reported having had a sexual health test over their lifetime (62.7%); however, only 56.6% had had an STI test within the past year. In total, 37.2% reported never having had a sexual health test. Qualitative responses provided similar themes as to why participants had never tested for HIV. These included, never having had sex, being currently sexually inactive, being in a monogamous relationship, sexual partners having already been tested, and considering themselves at a low or no risk were among the most common themes. Feeling uncomfortable and the psychological impacts of being misgendered and gender dysphoria were also listed as common reasons as to why participants had never had a sexual health test, as has been reported in previous research (Johnson, Nemeth, Mueller, Eliason, & Stuart, 2016; Poteat, et al., 2013). Some participants reported having been only tested for HIV for certain reasons such as surgery and job requirements. One participant shared that they had tested for HIV but not had a sexual health test as "other testing is not a priority and often uses gendered terms which makes me uncomfortable and avoidant".

Often sexual health screening guidelines are based on someone being symptomatic and then assessing the gender and sexuality of an individual to determine risk of exposure to STIs (Sevelius, Keatley, Calma, & Arnold, 2016). When it comes to diverse genders and sexualities, this may be difficult for sexual health clinicians who do not have thorough knowledge about diverse genders and sexualities to offer appropriate methods of testing (Torres et al., 2015). Participants in the TGD Needs Assessment were asked what sexual health tests they had received at their last sexual health appointment to ascertain if survey participants were being tested comprehensively (Positive Life NSW, et al., 2020). A blood test was the most common (51%) type of test participants received at their last sexual health screening, followed by a urine test (37.3%). Trans men were less likely to have had a blood test (45.3%) and trans women were less likely to report having a urine test (28.5%) compared to the other groups of participants.

Recently, substantial attention has been paid to pre-exposure prophylaxis (PrEP), as a biomedical HIV prevention intervention (Golub, Gamarel, Rendina, Surace, & Lelutiu-Weinberger, 2013). The first clinical trial of PrEP (the Chemoprophylaxis for HIV Prevention in Men study, also known as 'iPrEx') included high-risk MSM and trans women and found that PrEP reduced the risk of HIV acquisition by 44% (Grant et al., 2011). In the Positive Life Study, 69.8% of participants knew about PrEP, and 3.3% were currently taking it. Recently, substantial attention has been paid to pre-exposure prophylaxis (PrEP), as a biomedical HIV prevention intervention (Golub et al., 2013). The first clinical trial of PrEP (the Chemoprophylaxis for HIV Prevention in Men study, also known as 'iPrEx') included high-risk MSM and trans women and found that PrEP reduced the risk of HIV acquisition by 44% (Grant et al., 2011). In the TGD Needs Assessment, 54.7% of participants knew about PrEP, and 3% were currently taking it.

Experiences of negative interactions with HCPs related to sexual health can act as barriers to the use of PrEP, and to maintaining treatment adherence, with serious implications for the health and wellbeing of TGD people (Golub et al., 2013; Sevelius, et al., 2016).

"I'm scared of being judged": interactions with HCPs about sexual health

Health Professionals rarely understand the needs of Trans or Gender Non-conforming people's sexual health. A difficult conversation for someone who is cisgender becomes almost impossible to navigate when you are Trans.

(Sheehan, 2020)

HCPs are often reluctant to discuss sexuality with TGD patients, due to lack of knowledge or confidence (Snelgrove, Jasudavisius, Rowe, Head, & Bauer, 2012). In the TGD Needs Assessment, conversations about sexual health were most often initiated by participants themselves (61.25%), followed by their 'doctor' (33.3%), 'peers/friends' (20%), and 'partners' (19.5%). People who identified as gender diverse (assigned female at birth) were more likely to have their peers/friends and partners initiate a conversation about sexual health compared with other groups of participants. Trans men were more likely to have conversations about their sexual health initiated by their doctor than trans women or gender diverse participants.

Many participants reported feeling 'comfortable' or 'very comfortable' (45.9%) talking about sexual health with health professionals, followed by 'neither comfortable nor uncomfortable' (27.9%). Approximately one in four participants (26.1%) felt either 'uncomfortable' or 'very uncomfortable' discussing sexual health. Trans men and people who are gender diverse (assigned female at birth) were more likely to report feeling 'uncomfortable' which, in turn, might explain why these two participant groups were less likely themselves to initiate a conversation about sexual health with a healthcare provider (Positive Life NSW, et al., 2020).

Table 5.1 represents what would make the conversation about sexual health with healthcare providers more comfortable, using participants' (n=141) own words to highlight the most common themes.

Feeling unsafe is a significant barrier to TGD people discussing sexual health with HCPs (Poteat et al., 2013). When accessing sexual health services, most of the TGD Needs Assessment participants felt 'somewhat safe' (37.1%) and 'very safe' (22.8%). A further, 31.6% felt 'neither safe nor unsafe', 6.8% who felt 'unsafe', and 1.7% who felt 'very unsafe'. Trans men and people who are gender diverse (assigned female at birth) were more likely to report lower rates of feeling 'very safe' (17.3% and 15.2%, respectively) and higher rates of feeling 'unsafe' (10.3% and 10.9%, respectively).

Participants in the Positive Life Study were asked if they would like to share about their feelings of safety when accessing sexual health services. Participants indicated that many felt safer when accessing TGD inclusive or lesbian, gay, bisexual, transgender, queer and/or intersex (LGBTQI) clinics, and less safe and more uncomfortable in mainstream/non-LGBTQI clinics. Many participants reported feeling that they had to be the educator about TGD health to their healthcare providers. Others had concerns of stigma and discrimination, not being listened to, privacy issues, and assumptions by healthcare providers about their gender and sexuality.

TABLE 5.1 What would make the conversation about sexual health with healthcare providers more comfortable?

Health providers who are allies, respectful, and non-judgmental (n=48)
"Knowledge that my GP is an ally of the LGBTI community."
"Visible signs of support for LGBTQI patients."
"I am scared of being judged (about who I sleep with)."
"I'm often asked very probing questions that aren't medically relevant. I'm clearly a curiosity."

Health providers who don't make assumptions
"Not having doctors assume I use my body in particular ways. Letting me explain in my own words."
"Talking to us about our genitals they should ask first what we call it before they assume."
"Less heteronormativity in the assumptions they make about who I'm having sex with or the kinds of sex I have."

Health providers who are knowledgeable of trans and gender diverse care (n=20)
"Knowing the person is trained in gender affirming care."
"Medical professionals that have a better idea of what non-binary is and what it means."
"Knowing that the doctor will have at least some understanding of what it's like to relate to your own body and to have sex as a trans person."

Knowledge and comfort in talking about alternative and queer sexualities and ways of having sex (n=18)
"Understanding of alternative sexualities and ways of having sex."
"A greater understanding of queer sex and trans bodies."

Dysphoria and being comfortable with self (n=17)
"My dysphoria causes me to be uncomfortable talking about my 'junk'."
"It makes me feel dysphoric so I would rather avoid the topic."
"I'd just have to be more comfortable with myself."

Peers and queer doctors available for support (n=11)
"Queer doctors."
"Discussing the matter with professionals who have a more similar identity to my own."
"A doctor that is gay/understands queer people or is younger."

Understanding and using correct language/terminology (n=9)
"Being out as trans and the healthcare professional not gendering body parts/using the words I use for my body make me more comfortable."
"I have to start by explaining what my words mean and they often just don't understand."

If the health providers initiated conversations about sexual health (n=3)
"If they brought the conversation up and asked about screenings instead of having to request it for myself."
"If doctors were to casually ask if I would like a screening, that would be helpful. Initiating that kind of conversation is really hard to do."
"A doctor who asked to do the screening so I don't have to raise it."

Accessibility to sexual health services (n=3)
"Well-advertised and welcoming place so I can find them."
"I don't live in the right area and can't afford to move."
"I wouldn't speak with my GP. They get uncomfortable. When I go to the sexual health clinic though, doctors visit from Sydney and they are amazing, kind and understanding – I wish they were available every week – sometimes you need to wait a month to see one."

Another group of survey participants reported positive experiences when accessing sexual health services and many felt safe with their regular GP who they trusted and had built rapport with and who was respectful. Some reported feeling unsafe due to psychological distress associated with talking about bodies and sex, as well as uncertainty associated with whether they would be supported when visiting a new health professional. Feeling unsafe in encounters with HCPs is a manifestation of minority stress, the chronic and cumulative stress on those with stigmatised sexual and gender identities, associated with mental health outcomes (Mongelli et al., 2019). We will now turn to research on mental health in TGD communities, and the association of mental health with minority stress, including a discussion of the predictors of self-reported mental health and interactions with HCPs in the TGD Needs Assessment.

"Discrimination takes a toll": mental health and minority stress

LGBTQI (lesbian, gay, bisexual, transgender, queer and intersex) communities are more likely to be diagnosed and treated with mental health problems in comparison to the general population. For example, a recent Australian study reporting that 41% LGBTQI people aged 16 or over met the criteria for a mental health disorder, compared to 20% for the general population (Australian Bureau of Statistics (ABS), 2008; Leonard, Lyons, & Bariola, 2015). Research consistently highlights that compared to LGBQ and cis people, TGD individuals are more likely to experience mental health problems and have suicidal tendencies (Couch et al., 2007; Hyde, et al., 2014; Pflum, Testa, Balsam, Goldblum, & Bongar, 2015). A study of self-reported mental health in LGBTQ people found that TGD participants had the highest rate of mental health conditions, with 38.3% of trans men experiencing depression, and 42.6% experiencing anxiety, whilst 50% of trans women experienced depression and 34.4% experienced anxiety (Leonard et al., 2015). Another study highlighted that TGD individuals are four times as likely to be diagnosed with depression in their lifetime, and approximately one and a half times more likely to be diagnosed with anxiety, compared to the cisgender population (Hyde et al., 2014). These higher rates of distress experienced by TGD people are attributed to minority stress (Carmel & Erickson-Schroth, 2016; Ellis, Bailey, & McNeil, 2015). This includes stigma, social exclusion, and discrimination commonly associated with TGD and LGBQ identities (described as distal stressors), as well as negative self-beliefs and expectations of TGD and LGBQ people, including internalised transphobia and homophobia, concealment of identity, and stigma consciousness – vigilance and expectation of rejection in social interactions (described as proximal stressors) (Meyer, 2003; Morandini, Blaszczynski, Dar-Nimrod, & Ross, 2015).

TGD people experience discrimination in a range of settings, including healthcare, employment, and educational institutions (Hyde et al., 2014). For example, in a national Australian survey, nearly one in three TGD people reported experiencing at least one instance of discrimination and harassment, ranging from social exclusion to violence and assault (Hyde et al., 2014). In a study of young TGD people, 66% of the sample had experienced verbal abuse, while 21% had experienced physical abuse, and 32% experienced other forms of abuse and discrimination

(Smith et al., 2014). There are also reports of discrimination when trying to access healthcare, with the healthcare system failing to meet the needs of TGD individuals (Ellis et al., 2015; Hyde et al., 2014; Kerr et al., 2019; Kerr, Fisher, & Jones, 2021). Young trans people who had negative healthcare experiences reported more severe depressive symptoms, higher rates of other mental health disorders and increased rates of self-harm or attempted suicide (Strauss et al., 2020).

In the TGD Needs Assessment, we examined the association between self-reported mental health and discrimination in life, across a range of domains. Experiences of discrimination were common among participants, with 83% reporting experiencing discrimination in employment, education, healthcare, relationships, sexual connection, family, or housing. The most common area of discrimination experienced by participants was 'family' (38.1%). Trans men and people who are gender diverse (assigned female at birth) were more likely to report 'family' as an area of discrimination than the other two participant groups. 'Relationships' (33.8%), 'online' (33.5%), 'employment' (33.2%), and 'healthcare' (26.9%) were other areas of discrimination.

Self-reported mental health was reported to be 'very poor' or 'poor' for 39% of participants, 'OK' for 35.5%, and 'good' or 'very good' for 25.6%, consistent with the previous research that shows poor mental health in the TGD community (e.g., Hyde et al., 2014; Couch et al., 2007). When asked whether they had ever been diagnosed with mental health conditions, 62.2% reported depression, 59.1% anxiety, 21.3% post-traumatic stress disorder, 9.2% eating disorder, 7% personality disorder, and 3.6% psychosis, suggesting significant interaction with HCPs in relation to mental health concerns. Current self-reported mental health was significantly lower for those who reported more discrimination across several areas. This was in accordance with a minority stress framework, which predicts experiences of discrimination would accumulate and add to the psychological stress that TGD people experience (Carmel & Erickson-Schroth, 2016; Meyer, 2012).

In the qualitative analysis, participants described discrimination as varying from "misgendering", "bullying, sexual/physical harassment", to "systematic discrimination" and "micro aggressions". This was described as taking "a toll on mental health" as it can lead to feeling "isolated and unsupported", and to "a nervous breakdown". For those who did not report experiencing discrimination, it was due to "the privilege of passing", or "by having to remain stealth", with some saying they "decided to stay closeted due to fear". This choice also impacts mental health, with participants describing they have to "censor myself and that is mentally draining". It would also impact sense of self with one participant expressing they "pretend to be a man when I am not really a man. This impacts everything".

"The best thing I ever did": gender affirmation improves mental health and wellbeing

In the Positive Life Study, 62.9% of participants were taking gender affirming hormonal therapy (GAHT) and 25% had engaged in gender confirming surgery (GCS) (Positive Life NSW, et al., 2020), with engagement in GAHT or GAS found to be significant predictors of positive mental health (Sheehan, 2020). Gender affirmation is the process of an individual outwardly affirming and presenting as their true gender (Dalzell & Protos, 2020). Within TGD communities there is a high rate of body dislike or dysphoria pre gender affirmation, with one report highlighting that two thirds of their sample indicated a strong or moderate dislike for their bodies (Kerr, et al., 2019). For some TGD individuals, gender affirmation may be a way to help alleviate some of this bodily discomfort (Dalzell & Protos, 2020). In a 2019 report of 1,613 Australian TGD individuals aged 16-80, 79.9% of participants had undertaken action, either medical or non-medical, to alter their body to affirm their gender (Callander, et al., 2019). In a 2014 study of 189 young TGD people, 26% of participants had undertaken or were currently undertaking a medical gender affirmation (Smith, et al., 2014).

Medical affirmation involving GAHT or GCS facilitates development of secondary physical characteristics of gender, such as voice changes or tissue development. HCPs play a key role in medical gender affirmation. Previous research has also reported that access to GAHT improves quality of life and produces a marked difference in clinically significant depressive symptoms (Couch et al., 2007; Hyde et al., 2014; McNeil, Bailey, Ellis, Morton, & Regan, 2012). One study found that clinically relevant depressive symptoms were lowest for participants currently engaging in GAHT, and that, conversely, the highest level of clinically significant depressive symptoms were found for those who wanted GAHT but were not currently engaging in it (Hyde et al., 2014). Gender affirming surgery has also been found to be connected to physical health, with those having had GCS having higher rates of self-reported physical health (Riggs, Coleman, & Due, 2014). The positive impact that medical affirmation has on mental health may be due to a reduction in distress associated with gender dysphoria (White Hughto & Reisner, 2016). Medical affirmation also has the potential to reduce harassment, assisting an individual to have gender markers consistent with identified gender, allowing them to 'blend' or pass as cisgender (Rood et al., 2017; Ussher, Hawkey et al., 2022). However, the positive association between GHAT, GCS, and mental health is contingent upon the TGD person wanting to pursue medical affirmation (Hyde et al., 2014). As there are many different forms of affirmation, not every TGD person may want to undertake medical procedures to affirm their identity (Strauss et al., 2017).

In the qualitative findings of the TGD Needs Assessment, a common theme among participants that had surgical affirmation was an increase in sense of self, which "alleviated dysphoria", as the experience was "gender-affirming", and "liberating". One participant noted that "I'm so happy that my body is as close to a cismale body as I can currently get", with another highlighting that despite "years of gatekeeping … the actual surgery was lifesaving and best thing I ever did". The physical alignment with identified gender also appears to have a positive impact on mental health with a participant expressing becoming their "true me – after years of not addressing my gender dysphoria", and another emphasising that since having the surgeries their "mental health and wellbeing raised significantly and [I] experience a better quality of life". Other participants expressed feeling "content", and "complete" after having a form of surgical affirmation.

However, participants also noted accessibility issues around surgical affirmation, with "very few options" and "not enough experienced surgeons in the field in Australia", especially for those assigned female at birth. Those who found adequate HCPs and services reported extensive wait periods up to "4 months", and often followed by an extensive process which was "a humiliating waste of time to jump through hoops for approval". Participants also identified wanting support with the financial cost of services associated with being TGD, with the "cost of psychologist and doctors" adding up to be "financially crippling" for some participants so that "I can't afford the mental health services that I need".

Within Australia, access to any medical gender affirmation has historically been granted only after a diagnosis of gender dysphoria (Coleman et al., 2012; Lyons, 2017). This has changed with new Auspath guidelines which emphasise informed consent, and HCP support for gender affirmation without the need for pathologising diagnosis (AusPATH., 2022). For TGD people who may be entering the health system to pursue medical affirmation, HCPs can be viewed as gatekeepers who determine whether individuals should undertake medical procedures to affirm their gender (Ellis et al., 2015). HCPs are viewed as having the power to delay or deny access to GAHT, which can make it difficult to establish an authentic relationship between practitioner and client. This may explain the perceived negative experiences many TGD people report with psychiatrists and surgeons (Ellis et al., 2015; Riggs et al., 2014), and the association between mental health and comfort in discussions with healthcare professionals.

Mental health and interactions with healthcare professionals

In the TGD Needs Assessment, we examined the association between mental health and comfort in general healthcare, as well as comfort in discussing sexual health with clinicians. We found that comfort in healthcare settings, and comfort discussing sexual health, significantly predicted self-reported mental health, suggesting mental health was better for individuals who were more comfortable discussing sexual health with HCPs (Sheehan, 2020). This confirms previous research which found experiences with general practitioners influenced ratings of mental wellbeing for TGD people, with perceived discrimination resulting in lower ratings, whilst positive experiences, including greater comfort and respect, increased ratings of wellbeing (Riggs et al., 2014).

Accessing adequate healthcare can be a difficult and isolating experience for TGD individuals (Strauss et al., 2017). Healthcare needs can go unmet, with more than half of the participants in a recent study reporting that at some point in their life they did not receive healthcare when they felt they needed it (Kerr et al., 2019). Research has highlighted that harassment, discrimination, and HCP lack of awareness or understanding can be significant barriers to healthcare for TGD people (Wesp, Malcoe, Elliott, & Poteat, 2019). Many TGD people view HCPs to be ill informed about trans-related experiences and issues, and as a result feel uncomfortable discussing health concerns and needs, or feel required to educate HCPs, including on use of misgendering language (Riggs et al., 2014). Additionally, there is often concern about being pathologised, with general mental health issues being positioned by HCPs as a result of, or 'symptom' of being TGD (Ellis et al., 2015). Research has reported that experiences with psychiatrists and surgeons varies across the sex assigned at birth (Riggs, et al., 2014), with TGD people who were assigned male at birth rating their experience slightly better than those assigned female at birth. This difference may be indicative of availability of gender affirming surgery within Australia, with surgeries for TGD people assigned male at birth being more available than for those assigned female at birth. TGD people of colour report higher rates of discrimination than their white counterparts (Kattari, Walls, Whitfield, & Langenderfer-Magruder, 2015), reflecting the intersection of gender and cultural identities in experiences of minority stress.

"We need to be heard, respected and supported": misgendering and judgement by healthcare professionals

In the TGD Needs Assessment, positive experiences with HCPs involved them being helpful, caring, knowledgeable, and professional, whilst negative experiences included perceived intrusive or offensive questions. One participant noted that a "lack of services comes from a lack of education from professionals". Experiences with HCP commonly involved "misgendering", misnaming, and inadequately knowledgeable professionals. It was explained that "clinicians will misgender me, attribute my mental illness to being transgender, treat me poorly ... ask inappropriate questions". Participants expressed dissatisfaction due to difficulty accessing TGD-friendly health professionals, which will not "pass on judgement and verbal harm", or that are not "overflowing" with large wait periods because "there is not enough services across the board". Many survey participants emphasised they would be more comfortable in healthcare settings with "more knowledge among doctors, nurses, and reception staff on how to treat and address TGD patients", and "competent doctors who won't misgender you" – doctors who show "openness and acceptance" and have "forms asking for preferred name/pronouns" or "directly being asked". This will make the experience more "comfortable" so patients "don't have to hide things" but feel "heard, respected, listened to, supported".

Another common element was the want for HCPs to have better expertise and be knowledgeable about TGD health to ensure that doctors are "proactive about my health, that would do research", or "open about their experience ... and willing to accept my research where their own is lacking". Some participants expressed they would feel better with more accessible LGBTI services or "indications that the practice is LGBTI friendly", and that TGD people are "welcomed at the clinic through visible notices such as a sticker or poster". It should also include an "inclusive space" such as "gender neutral bathrooms". Many participants expressed healthcare can "trigger dysphoria", so a trained professional who has "less heteronormativity in the assumptions they make", or "with professionals who have a more similar identity to my own" in terms of sexuality, age, and race would be more comforting. However, other participants expressed that "TGD people have experiences that are unique from the rest of the LGBTQ community, but we are lumped in with LGBTQ which are inadequate in catering to trans needs".

"I wish I had known my options": absence of TGD specific resources and services

Overall, participants in the TGD Needs Assessment reported dissatisfaction in relation to availability of TGD-specific resources and services and said there were barriers to feeling comfortable and accessing necessary services. Most survey participants noted a lack of information and awareness of TGD people and their concerns, and that information on gender diversity, affirmation, and services available "came from friends in a very ad hoc way". It was also highlighted that these "resources are only available in a select few languages", and with participants asking not to "overlook intersectionality", including race and "disability". One participant noted a "lack of resources to inform me of how to begin the process" of affirmation, and another expressed "I just wish I had known my options in the first place". There was also a reported "lack of adequate services to deal with the ton of suicides and mental health problems facing TGD (people), especially in rural areas", and that a "lack of support in early transition leads to destructive/harmful behaviours …".

There were identifiable gaps within support services available to TGD people, which participants requested to be filled, including services "for partners of trans people", for family members, for non-binary individuals, for "those with mental health problems or substance users", for those "post-transition", in "regional Australia", and those older in age, as some expressed there is "a lot of support for young trans but not older trans people".

Conclusion

Equitable access to sexual health services is a human rights issue for TGD people. Sexual and reproductive justice requires that TGD people should feel safe and comfortable when seeking healthcare, and should be treated with dignity and respect by clinicians (Riggs & Bartholomaeus, 2020). This is not solely with an aim to improve sexual health – our analysis demonstrates that this has direct implications for mental health and wellbeing. The findings of the Positive Life/Gender Centre Inc/TGD Advisory Group TGD Needs Assessment confirm that the mental health of TGD individuals is influenced by discrimination and discomfort in interactions with HCPs, and ameliorated by gender affirmation. There needs to be education of general and sexual HCPs of the needs and concerns of TGD people (Torres et al., 2015), with TGD inclusive practices being universally offered. Intersecting identities which may increase vulnerability need to be acknowledged, including the intersection of being TGD, sexuality diversity, and diverse cultural background (Wesp et al., 2019). There needs to be support for gender affirmation through hormones or surgery, if this is what a person wants (White Hughto & Reisner, 2016). As gender affirmation has implications for friends and family (Charter, Ussher, Perz, & Robinson, 2022), it is important to have information and support services available to assist everyone involved. The Informed Consent (IC) model for gender affirmation from the World Professional Association for Transgender Health (2012) has been evaluated positively by TGD people (Pallotta-Chiarolli, Wiggins, & Locke, 2019), alongside other TGD affirmative care, including use of correct pronouns, staff trained in cultural safety, non-gendered bathroom facilities, and trans and gender diverse specific literature and health resources (Arora et al., 2020). The meaning and experience of sexual health for TGD people needs to be considered when developing programs of support and intervention. Finally, to ensure that sexual health policy and support services meet the needs of TGD people, it is critical that TGD people are at the centre of leadership, program, and policy development. Only then will we have a situation of sexual and reproductive justice for TGD communities.

Trans and Gender Diverse Expert Advisory Group

Jett Black, Imogen Brackin, Teddy Cook, Dash Gray, Camryn Hicks, Natasha Io, Chantell Martin, Rachel Smith. Without the advisory group this work would not have been possible.

Acknowledgements

Positive Life, The Gender Centre Inc. and the Trans and Gender Diverse (TGD) Expert Advisory Group would like to thank the trans and gender diverse people across Australia who took the time to respond to this survey and share their knowledge and experience freely.

Note

1 The TGD advisory group of the study reported in this chapter prefer to use the acronym TGD (trans and gender diverse) to describe the population being discussed. We use this acronym throughout the chapter.

References

Australian Bureau of Statistics (ABS). (2008). National Survey of Mental Health and Wellbeing. Summary of results, 2007. Retrieved from www.abs.gov.au/ausstats/abs@.nsf/productsbytitle/3F8A5DFCBECAD9C0CA2568A900139380?OpenDocument

Arora, M., Walker, K., Luu, J., Duvivier, R. J., Dune, T., & Wynne, K. (2020). Education of the medical profession to facilitate delivery of transgender health care in an Australian health district. *Australian Journal of Primary Health*, *26*(1), 17–23.

AusPATH. (2022). *Australian informed consent standards of care for gender affirming hormone therapy*, from https://auspath.org.au/2022/03/31/auspath-australian-informed-consent-standards-of-care-for-gender-affirming-hormone-therapy/

Australian Government Department of Health. (2018a). *Eighth national HIV strategy 2018–2022*. Retrieved October 8, 2019, from www1.health.gov.au/internet/main/publishing. nsf/Content/ohp-bbvs-1/$File/HIV-Eight-Nat-Strategy-2018a-22.pdf

Australian Government Department of Health. (2018b). *Fourth national sexually transmissible infections strategy*. Retrieved October 8, 2019, from www1.health.gov.au/internet/main/ publishing.nsf/Content/ohp-bbvs-1/$File/STI-Fourth-Nat-Strategy-2018b-22.pdf

Balik, C. H. A., Bilgin, H., Uluman, O. T., Sukut, O., Yilmaz, S., & Buzlu, S. (2020). A systematic review of the discrimination against sexual and gender minority in health care settings. *International Journal of Health Services*, *50*(1), 44–61.

Baral, S. D. D., Poteat, T. P., Strömdahl, S. M. D., Wirtz, A. L. M. H. S., Guadamuz, T. E. P., & Beyrer, C. P. (2013). Worldwide burden of HIV in transgender women: a systematic review and meta-analysis. *The Lancet Infectious Diseases*, *13*(3), 214–222.

Callander, D., Wiggins, J., Rosenberg, S., Cornelisse, V. J., Duck-Chong, E., Holt, M., … Cook, T. (2019). *The 2018 Australian trans and gender diverse sexual health survey: Report of findings*. Sydney, NSW: The Kirby Institute.

Carmel, T. C., & Erickson-Schroth, L. (2016). Mental health and the transgender population. *Journal of Psychosocial Nursing and Mental Health Services*, *54*(12), 44–48.

Charter, R., Ussher, J. M., Perz, J., & Robinson, K. H. (2022). Transgender parents: Negotiating "coming out" and gender affirmation with children and co-parents. *Journal of Homosexuality*, *3*, 1–23.

Clements-Nolle, K., Marx, R., Guzman, R., & Katz, M. (2001). HIV prevalence, risk behaviors, health care use, and mental health status of transgender persons: Implications for public health intervention. *American Journal of Public Health (1971)*, *91*(6), 915–921.

Coleman, E., Bockting, W., Botzer, M., Cohen-Kettenis, P., DeCuypere, G., Feldman, J., … Zucker, K. (2012). Standards of care for the health of transsexual, transgender, and gender-nonconforming people, version 7. *International Journal of Transgenderism*, *13*(4), 165–232.

Couch, M., Pitts, M., Mulcare, H., Croy, S., Mitchell, A., & Patel, S. (2007). *TranZnation – a report on the health and wellbeing of transgendered people in Australia and New Zealand*. Melbourne: Australian Research Centre in Sex, Health and Society, LaTrobe University.

Dalzell, H., & Protos, K. (2020). *A clinician's guide to gender identity and body image: Practical support for working with transgender and gender-expansive clients*. London: Jessica Kingsley.

Ellis, S. J., Bailey, L., & McNeil, J. (2015). Trans people's experiences of mental health and gender identity services: A UK study. *Journal of Gay & Lesbian Mental Health*, *19*(1), 4–20.

Golub, S. A., Gamarel, K. E., Rendina, H. J., Surace, A., & Lelutiu-Weinberger, C. L. (2013). From efficacy to effectiveness: Facilitators and barriers to PrEP acceptability and motivations for adherence among MSM and transgender women in New York City. *AIDS Patient Care STDS*, *27*(4), 248–254.

Grant, J., Keisling, M., Harrison, J., Mottet, L., Herman, J., & Tanis, J. (2011). *Injustice at Every Turn: A Report of the National Transgender Discrimination Survey*.

Hyde, Z., Doherty, M., Tilley, P., McCaul, K., Rooney, R., & Jancey, J. (2014). *The First Australian National Trans Mental Health Study: Summary of results*. Perth: School of Public Health, Curtin University.

James, S. E., Herman, J. L., Rankin, S., Keisling, M., Mottet, L., & Anafi, M. (2016). *The Report of the 2015 U.S. Transgender Survey*. In N. C. F. T. Equality (Ed.). Washington, DC.

Jasek, E., Chow, E. P., Ong, J. J., Bradshaw, C. S., Chen, M. Y., Hocking, J. S., … Fairley, C. K. (2017). Sexually transmitted infections in Melbourne, Australia from 1918 to

2016: Nearly a century of data. *Communicable Diseases Intelligence Quarterly Report, 41*(3), E212–E222.

Johnson, M. J., Nemeth, L. S., Mueller, M., Eliason, M. J., & Stuart, G. W. (2016). Qualitative study of cervical cancer screening among lesbian and bisexual women and transgender men. *Cancer Nursing, 39*(6), 455–463.

Kattari, S. K., Walls, N. E., Whitfield, D. L., & Langenderfer-Magruder, L. (2015). Racial and ethnic differences in experiences of discrimination in accessing health services among transgender people in the United States. *The International Journal of Transgenderism, 16*(2), 68–79.

Kerr, L., Fisher, C., & Jones, T. (2019). *TRANScending discrimination in health & cancer care: A study of trans & gender diverse Australians.* ARCSHS Monograph Series No. 117. Melbourne: La Trobe University.

Kerr, L., Fisher, C. M., & Jones, T. (2021). "I'm not from another planet": The alienating cancer care experiences of trans and gender-diverse people. *Cancer Nursing, 1*(6), E438–446.

Leonard, W., Lyons, A., & Bariola, E. (2015). *A closer look at private lives 2: Addressing the mental health and wellbeing of lesbian, gay, bisexual, and transgender (LGBT) Australians.* Melbourne: Australian Research Centre in Sex, Health and Society, La Trobe University.

Lyons, A. (2017). Journey to care. *Good Practice, 4,* from www.racgp.org.au/download/Documents/Good%20Practice/2017/April/GP2017-april-transgender-patients-journey-to-care.pdf

McNeil, J., Bailey, L., Ellis, S., Morton, J., & Regan, M. (2012). *Trans mental health study 2012.* Retrieved from www.scottishtrans.org/wp-content/uploads/2013/03/trans_mh_study.pdf

Meyer, D. (2012). An intersectional analysis of lesbian, gay, bisexual, and transgender (LGBT) people's evaluations of anti-queer violence. *Gender & Society, 26*(6), 849–873.

Meyer, I. H. (2003). Prejudice, social stress, and mental health in lesbian, gay, and bisexual populations: Conceptual issues and research evidence. *Psychological Bulletin, 129,* 674–697.

Mongelli, F., Perrone, D., Balducci, J., Sacchetti, A., Ferrari, S., Mattei, G., & Galeazzi, G. M. (2019). Minority stress and mental health among LGBT populations: An update on the evidence. *Minerva Psichiatrica, 60*(1), 27–50.

Morandini, J. S., Blaszczynski, A., Dar-Nimrod, I., & Ross, M. W. (2015). Minority stress and community connectedness among gay, lesbian and bisexual Australians: A comparison of rural and metropolitan localities. *Australian and New Zealand Journal of Public Health, 39*(3), 260–266.

Pallotta-Chiarolli, M., Wiggins, J., & Locke, P. (2019). *"We need much more of the same": An evaluation of equinox gender diverse health centre.* Melbourne: Thorne Harbour Health.

Pflum, S. R., Testa, R. J., Balsam, K. F., Goldblum, P. B., & Bongar, B. (2015). Social support, trans community connectedness, and mental health symptoms among transgender and gender nonconforming adults. *Psychology of Sexual Orientation and Gender Diversity, 2*(3), 281–286.

Pitts, M., Smith, A., Mitchell, A., & Patel, S. (2006). *Private lives: A report on the health and wellbeing of GLBTI Australians.* Melbourne: Australian Research Centre in Sex, Health and Society, La Trobe University.

Positive Life NSW, The Gender Centre Inc., & TGD Expert Advisory Group. (2020). *Trans and gender diverse people health and social needs assessment: A community survey.* Retrieved from https://apo.org.au/node/310630

Poteat, T., German, D., & Kerrigan, D. (2013). Managing uncertainty: A grounded theory of stigma in transgender health care encounters. *Social Science and Medicine, 84,* 22–29.

Riggs, D. W., & Bartholomaeus, C. (2020). Toward trans reproductive justice: A qualitative analysis of views on fertility preservation for Australian transgender and non-binary people. *Journal of Social Issues*, *76*(2), 314–337.

Riggs, D. W., Coleman, K., & Due, C. (2014). Healthcare experiences of gender diverse Australians: A mixed-methods, self-report survey. *BMC Public Health*, *14*(1), 230–230.

Rood, B. A., Maroney, M. R., Puckett, J. A., Berman, A. K., Reisner, S. L., & Pantalone, D. W. (2017). Identity concealment in transgender adults: A qualitative assessment of minority stress and gender affirmation. *American Journal of Orthopsychiatry*, *87*(6), 704–713.

Seelman, K. L., Colón-Diaz, M. J. P., LeCroix, R. H., Xavier-Brier, M., & Kattari, L. (2017). Transgender noninclusive healthcare and delaying care because of fear: Connections to general health and mental health among transgender adults. *Transgender Health*, *2*(1), 17–28.

Sevelius, J. M., Keatley, J., Calma, N., & Arnold, E. (2016). "I am not a man": Trans-specific barriers and facilitators to PrEP acceptability among transgender women. *Global Public Health*, *11*(7–8), 1060–1075.

Sheehan, C. (2020). *Mitigating mental health: Influences of discrimination, comfort in healthcare settings and affirmation on transgender and gender diverse individuals* Masters of Clinical Psychology, Western Sydney University, unpublished Master's thesis.

Shires, D. A., & Jaffee, K. (2015). Factors associated with health care discrimination experiences among a national sample of female-to-male transgender individuals. *Health & social work*, *40*(2), 134–141.

Smith, E., Jones, T., Ward, R., Dixon, J., Mitchell, A., & Hillier, L. (2014). *From blues to rainbows: Mental health and wellbeing of gender diverse and transgender young people in Australia*. Melbourne: The Australian Research Centre in Sex, Health, and Society.

Snelgrove, J. W., Jasudavisius, A. M., Rowe, B. W., Head, E. M., & Bauer, G. R. (2012). "Completely out-at-sea" with "two-gender medicine": A qualitative analysis of physician-side barriers to providing healthcare for transgender patients. *BMC Health Services Research*, *12*(1), 110–110.

Stephens, S. C., Bernstein, K. T., & Philip, S. S. (2010). Male to female and female to male transgender persons have different sexual risk behaviors yet similar rates of STDs and HIV. *AIDS and Behavior*, *15*(3), 683–686.

Strauss, P., Cook, A., Winter, S., Watson, V., Wright Toussaint, D., & Lin, A. (2017). *Trans pathways: The mental health experiences and care pathways of trans young people*. Summary of results: Perth, Australia: Telethon Kids Institute.

Strauss, P., Cook, A., Winter, S., Watson, V., Wright Toussaint, D., & Lin, A. (2020). Associations between negative life experiences and the mental health of trans and gender diverse young people in Australia: Findings from Trans Pathways. *Psychological Medicine*, *50*(5), 808–817.

Torres, C. G., Renfrew, M., Kenst, K., Tan-McGrory, A., Betancourt, J. R., & López, L. (2015). Improving transgender health by building safe clinical environments that promote existing resilience: Results from a qualitative analysis of providers. *BMC Pediatrics*, *15*(187), 187–187.

UNAIDS. (2015). UNAIDS 2016–2021 *Strategy: On the fast-track to end AIDS*. Retrieved October 8, 2019, from www.unaids.org/sites/default/files/media_asset/20151027_UNAIDS_PCB37_15_18_EN_rev1.pdf

Ussher, J. M., Allison, K., Perz, J., Power, R., & The Out with Cancer Study Team. (2022a). LGBTQI cancer patients' quality of life and distress: A comparison by gender, sexuality, age, cancer type and geographical remoteness. *Frontiers in Oncology*, doi.org/10.3389/fonc.2022.873642

Ussher, J. M., Hawkey, A., Perz, J., Liamputtong, P., Sekar, J., Marjadi, B., ... Brook, E. (2022b). Crossing boundaries and fetishization: Experiences of sexual violence for trans women of color. *Journal of Interpersonal Violence*, *37*(5–6), NP3552–NP3584.

Wesp, L. M., Malcoe, L. H., Elliott, A., & Poteat, T. (2019). Intersectionality research for transgender health justice: A theory-driven conceptual framework for structural analysis of transgender health inequities. *Transgender Health*, *4*(1), 287–296.

White Hughto, J. M., & Reisner, S. L. (2016). A systematic review of the effects of hormone therapy on psychological functioning and quality of life in transgender individuals. *Transgender Health*, *1*(1), 21–31.

World Health Organization. (2015). *Policy brief: Transgender people and HIV*. Retrieved from https://apps.who.int/iris/bitstream/handle/10665/179517/WHO_HIV_2015.17_eng.pdf

World Professional Association for Transgender Health. (2012). *Standards of care for the health of transsexual, transgender, and gendernonconforming people, SOC 7*. Retrieved from www.wpath.org/media/cms/Documents/SOC%20v7/Standards%20of%20Care_V7%20Full%20Book_English.pdf

6

HOLISTIC SEXUALITY EDUCATION AND FERTILITY COUNSELLING FOR TRANS CHILDREN AND YOUNG PEOPLE

Kerry H. Robinson, Cristyn Davies, Jane M. Ussher and Rachel Skinner

Introduction

Sexuality education is core to providing critical foundational information for children's and young people's sexual health and wellbeing, and sexual citizenship (Robinson, 2022). However, sexuality education is fundamentally a political field, especially in the context of children and young people. Sexuality education in schools is highly contentious, resulting in social, cultural, and educational regulations restricting children's and young people's access to this knowledge. In many countries, regulations prevail about what is included in the sexuality education curriculum in schools, at what age this information can be accessed – both formally and informally in schools and the home – and who should be educating children and young people about sex and sexuality.

Some adults consider aspects of sexuality education as age 'inappropriate' for children and young people. These topics can include discussions on desire, young people's agency as gendered and sexual subjects, contraception, abortion, and gender and sexuality diversity (Robinson, Smith & Davies, 2017). Dominant discourses of childhood and sexuality are foundational to the controversial nature of sex and sexuality education and underpin the strict regulation of children's and young people's access to this knowledge, resulting from its constitution as 'adults only' information. These socio-cultural barriers prevent children and young people from accessing relevant sex and sexuality education throughout their early lives, both in schools and in families, potentially impacting their short and longer-term health and wellbeing (Robinson, 2013; Robinson, Smith & Davies, 2017; Shannon, 2022).

Trans children and young people are particularly impacted by these restrictive socio-cultural barriers and lack of access to relevant sexuality education. For these young people, sex and sexuality education, framed within binary gender discourses, can be a stressful and anxiety-provoking aspect of their early schooling

DOI: 10.4324/9781003138310-6

experiences. In sexuality education classes in co-educational schools, young people are often divided by binary gender, and topics discussed relate to the perceived needs of the respective genders. Consequently, many trans young people do not receive sexuality education pertinent to their needs (Riggs & Bartholomaeus, 2018; Shannon, 2022). This is inequitable as many trans young people are required to make significant decisions about their future reproductive lives, family formations, fertility preservation, and future relationships, or about the gender of future partners – when they are making decisions about gender-affirming hormones. Access to 'holistic' sexuality education and fertility counselling is important for trans young people to be informed about their bodies, future reproductive options, fertility, fertility preservation, and any associated risks (Lai et al., 2021; Lai et al., 2020; Pang et al., 2020). Fertility education is generally poorly addressed in sexuality education in schools for all young people. For trans young people, the lack of access to relevant information and education can lead to significant health inequities.

The discussion in this chapter is informed not just by the published literature relevant to sexuality education, fertility, and the reproductive futures of trans children and young people, but also by the findings from two Australian research projects conducted by the authors. Important issues related to trans children's and young people's access to sexuality education are addressed, including: sexuality education in schools; education/counselling about fertility, reproductive futures, and fertility preservation; and the role of sexuality education in building sexual citizenship early in life. We also address the socio-cultural barriers associated with age and childhood that not only prevent access to holistic sexuality education for all children and young people, but also impact some adults' perceptions of children's abilities to make important decisions about their lives.

What is holistic sexuality education?

Sexuality education in this chapter is inclusive of a broad range of understandings of sex and sexuality education, such as sexual health education, sex and relationships education, inclusive sexuality education, genders and sexualities education, health and wellbeing education, and comprehensive sexuality education. While these terms are used in different contexts globally, in this chapter, sexuality education includes all aspects of sex, sexuality, gender, relationships, relevant to cisgender, trans, and non-binary people, and is inclusive of all sexualities. To reflect this, we consider 'holistic sexuality education' best captures inclusive sexuality education (European Expert Group on Sexuality Education, 2016). According to the *Standards for Sexuality Education in Europe* the concept of 'holistic sexuality education' is defined as:

> Learning about the cognitive, emotional, social, interactive and physical aspects of sexuality. Sexuality education starts early in childhood and

progresses through adolescence and adulthood. It aims at supporting and protecting sexual development. It gradually equips and empowers children and young people with information, skills and positive values to understand and enjoy their sexuality, have safe and fulfilling relationships and take responsibility for their own and other people's sexual health and well-being.

(WHO, 2010)

Holistic sexuality education acknowledges that this learning is not confined to schools. This education also needs to occur in families, health settings, and non-government organisations that work with young people. Holistic sexuality education also recognises that this learning is a process of lifelong learning, not a just one-off discussion, demonstrating that the sexual health needs of young people can change across their lives. Ultimately, sexuality education that meets the needs of all children and young people is a human right and key to the development of their sexual citizenship (Robinson, 2022).

The impact of the controversial nature of sexuality education in schools

Although sexual narratives saturate young people's lives from an early age, they have limited access to knowledge or discussions about gender, relationships, sex, sexuality, and reproductive futures, throughout their schooling. Instead, children's and young people's sexuality education is plagued with tensions and controversies, largely due to social anxieties stemming from cultural discourses that these issues are irrelevant, developmentally inappropriate, risky, and dangerous to young people, particularly pre-pubescent children (Robinson, 2013; Robinson, Smith & Davies, 2017). This is despite the demonstrated value of sexuality education to young people's health and wellbeing, which supports and builds informed decision making, including about their reproductive futures.

All children and young people should have access to relevant holistic sexuality education which starts early and continues throughout their lives. However, the sexuality education experiences of most children and young people are far from holistic or relevant; this is especially so for trans children and young people and those who are sexuality diverse. This is especially problematic as research has shown that SSAGQ (Same-sex attracted and gender questioning) young people are less likely to use a condom, twice as likely to become pregnant and more likely to contract a sexually transmitted infection (STI), and more likely to be sexually active at an earlier age compared to their cisgender and/or heterosexual peers (Hillier et al., 2010, p. ix and also chapter 4). Most research on sexuality education and young people has focused on heterosexual and cisgender young people, and to a much lesser extent, sexuality diverse young people's experiences, and is generally framed within discourses of risk and danger. Research on trans young people's perspectives and experiences of sexuality education have been limited. However, research has acknowledged and critiqued the lack of relevant information for trans young people in sexuality education and the cisgender heteronormative nature of this curriculum in schools (Robinson & Davies, 2008; Riggs, 2013; Bartholomaeus & Riggs, 2017; Owen, 2017; Robinson & Davies, 2017).

In Australia, sexuality education appears in the health and physical education curricula. However, access to sexuality education varies across Australian states and territories, schools, and individual classrooms. There is no guarantee that young people receive sexuality education to any great extent in their schooling, as it is not compulsory in most Australian jurisdictions, and what is taught is often determined by individual teachers and schools. Despite some acknowledgement in sexuality education curricula of the need to address lesbian, gay, bisexual, trans, and queer (LGBTQ+) issues, this does not always transfer to classroom discussions. In some schools, it is optional or required to have parental permission to participate in sexuality education classes. Some Australian jurisdictions regulate the inclusion of LGBTQ+ issues and discussions in sexuality education or in other curriculum areas through policies such as the 'Controversial Issues' policy (NSW Department of Education, 2021). In the state of New South Wales the Controversial Issues in School Policy require the identification and management of issues considered controversial; and require that parents or carers are aware of such activities and given the option of withdrawing their child from these sessions. The subjective nature of what is considered a controversial issue, not defined in the policy, can shift from school to school, principal to principal, teacher to teacher, and across parent communities. This approach to LGBTQ+ issues is a result of a long-term conservative political movement that has instigated moral panic about including trans and non-binary issues in particular, as well as sexuality diversity, in children's and young people's education (Ferfolja & Ullman, 2021; Robinson, 2012, 2013).

Controversy about sexuality education is not confined to Australia but reflects a recent global phenomenon focused on the exclusion of trans, non-binary, and sexuality diversity issues in school education across all sectors (e.g., Trump's Administration in the United States (Lopez, 2017); and Parental Rights Bill 2020 in Australia (McGowan, 2022)). Still, there has been considerable pushback from trans communities, their allies, and human rights advocates to defeat these attempts at undermining the rights of trans students, with some positive results. For example, the Biden Administration in the United States has revoked the Trump Administration's legislation undermining the rights of trans students to an inclusive, safe and discrimination-free education. Further, the Relationships Education, Relationships and Sex Education (RSE) and Health Education new guideline recommendations in the United Kingdom include teaching about LGBT issues. This will be mandatory in secondary schools but not in primary schools (Terence Higgins Trust, 2019). The recent introduction of the new Sex and Relationships Education in Wales is unquestionably one of the most holistic, radical, and inclusive curriculums globally. This curriculum is mandated for all children, includes addressing gender and sexuality diversity, and does not allow parents to withdraw their children for these classes. How more conservative families and community members adhere to these requirements is yet to be seen.

Trans young people, sexuality education, and fertility counselling: a review of the literature

Trans young people and sexuality education

Over the last decade, information regarding trans young people's experiences of sexuality education has been most often found in school climate reports on the safety and inclusion experiences of LGBTQ+ young people (Kosciw et al., 2020; Hillier et al., 2010). Over this time, research has shown that trans young people can complete their schooling without being provided with any sexuality education; that the sexuality education they do receive is most often not inclusive of trans and/or sexuality-diverse issues, is considered irrelevant, does not meet their needs regarding relationships, safe-sex practices, fertility, or reproductive futures, and comes way too late in their schooling (Hillier et al., 2010; Smith et al. 2014; Robinson, Smith & Davies, 2017; Shannon, 2022). These experiences were especially the case for transgender and gender-diverse young people (Smith et al. 2014).

Barrie Shannon's (2022) recent research on the sexuality education experiences of trans (aged 18–26) in Australia shows that not much has changed in the past decade or more. Overall, trans young people's experiences of sexuality education are still 'unengaging, irrelevant and alienating' (p. 109). Their experiences continue to be ignored and absent from most discussions in sexuality education in many schools. However, when they were included, it was rarely in a positive light, and in some cases the information provided is misinformation. Sexuality education for some participants in Shannon's research was segregated by binary gender and framed within the discourse of abstinence. One trans masculine young person in Shannon's study, Javier, reported the negative physical, emotional, and social impacts they experienced from the poor standard of sex education received at school:

> If sexual health was taught earlier, was non-segregated, was more inclusive and relevant, I could have avoided situations that effectively damaged my physical and emotional health, and I could have been given the tools to deal with being a victim of both prejudice and sexual assault … A better sex education program would have made me feel like I wasn't completely alone and would have prompted me to seek vital help from a much earlier age.
>
> *(Shannon, 2022, pp. 95–96)*

Javier was not only resentful about not receiving the practical sexual health information he required during his schooling, but also resented the symbolic violence implicit in silencing queer issues in the classroom. Trans young people reported that teachers lacked training in sexuality education, especially on trans and sexuality diversity issues, which increased their frustration and fuelled their anxieties in sexuality education classrooms. The following table shows what trans participants in Shannon's study (2022), identified as crucial elements of a trans positive sexuality education.

TABLE 6.1 Elements of trans positive sexuality education

Elements of trans positive sexuality education
Validation of trans identities and those of queer young people
Demystifying what it means to be trans
Sex-positive approach (not dominated by discourses of procreation and danger)
Sex, sexuality and relationships as fluid, fun, erotic, playful and romantic
Negotiating sexuality, relationships, and identity
Normalisation of queer families
Masculinities and femininities and queerness as social phenomena
Social media and advertising in young people's lives
Sexting
Critique of gender norms
Safe sex practices with any partner
Sexual consent/negotiating respectful relationships and sex with others
Sex beyond heterosexual intercourse
Non-judgemental discussions of porn, masturbation, and physical pleasure
Less scientific approach to sexual health information
Access to medical advice
No animated videos on reproduction, pregnancy and childbirth, puberty, body hair, and menstruation

Fertility and reproductive futures

An important part of sexuality education for young trans people includes information about fertility, future partners, family formations, and future reproductive possibilities. However, as pointed out previously, there are no discussions of these issues relevant to trans young people included in sexuality education in schools. There is limited research on how trans young people perceive their reproductive futures, including fertility preservation. The research to date that includes young people's perspectives on fertility, fertility preservation, and their reproductive futures highlights several important areas: (i) the role of parents in their decision making; (ii) factors that inhibit trans young people's choices to access fertility preservation options; (iii) young people's poor understandings of reproductive biology; (iv) the different priorities that trans young people have in their lives; and (v) young trans people's lack of engagement in discussions about fertility and fertility preservation in their early lives.

Research shows that parents play a significant role in trans young people's choices to undertake fertility preservation. Strang et al. (2018) explored 25 13–19 years old trans young people's perspectives of their reproductive futures. This US-based research also included a parent of each of the young people participating. Sixty-five per cent (65%) of parents hoped their children would have their own children; with 21% indicating they would be disappointed if their child did not have a genetically related child. Although Australian research conducted by Riggs and Bartholomaeus (2020) on trans young people's reproductive futures did not include children, it nonetheless pointed out that some parents encouraged children to undertake fertility preservation and had strong desires for their children to have genetically related children. This research involved three different qualitative studies, one with parents of trans children, the second with trans adults, and the third with healthcare professionals. Riggs and Bartholomaeus found parents were often concerned about compounding their child's dysphoria if encouraging or discussing fertility preservation with their children. They also pointed out that there was a strong pronatalist discourse directed towards those assumed female at birth (see also Chapter 8 in this book).

Although many trans young people wish to become parents, they may also have other priorities in their lives. Research conducted by Chiniara et al. (2019) with trans young people aged 12–18 years and their parents explored their perspectives on fertility and parenthood. This research asked participants to rank *having children* compared with other life priorities today and in ten years time. Almost all the trans young people ranked *having children* the lowest among eight life priorities today and in ten years, though it did increase in importance in the projected ten year outcomes for those trans young people who were presumed female at birth. Young people ranked good health, doing well in school/work, and having close friends as the highest priorities today and in ten-year projections. While it is possible that young people may change their minds about their priorities ten years hence, just as adults might, this does not invalidate the decisions they make today, drawing on the best available information (Pang, Giordano, Sood, & Skinner, 2021). Parents had similar rankings to those of their children. This latter point reinforces findings in other research reporting that parents have similar views on fertility and fertility preservation to their children (Lawlis, Donkin, Bates, Britto, & Conard, 2017; Walton-Betancourth et al., 2018).

There are key barriers that young trans people identify inhibiting their uptake of fertility preservation. Research in the Netherlands by Brik et al. (2018) with 35 trans girls reported several barriers including: not wanting to have children; wanting to adopt; feeling uncomfortable with masturbation or aversion to their penis; and being uncomfortable about being a biological father. Chen et al. (2017) explored the attitudes toward fertility and reproductive health among 156 trans and gender non-conforming adolescents aged 14–17 years in the United States. Almost half of these young people were interested in having children in the future, but most (75%) were interested in adoption rather than biological parenthood. Young people presumed female at birth were significantly more interested in adoption than those presumed male at birth; with more gender non-conforming young people interested in biological parenting than trans young people. Further, this study raised several other concerns reported by young people related to fertility and family formation, including: stigma toward same-gender maternal parenting; societal expectations; the impact of gender-affirming hormones on fertility; the expense of fertility preservation; gender dysphoria or discomfort; general concerns about pregnancy and parenting related to gender identities, such as pain, financial issues, and pre-existing health conditions impacting fertility (e.g. endometriosis). A study by Nehata, Tishelman, Caltabellotta, & Quinn (2017) also highlighted trans young people's preference for adoption, and raised similar concerns about feeling uncomfortable producing a sperm sample through masturbation, that fertility preservation was too expensive, as well as having concerns about potentially needing to delay hormone treatment. Fertility costs and invasiveness and discomfort associated with the procedures were also reinforced in Chiniara et al.'s (2019) research. Nehata et al. (2017) suggest that more research is needed to ascertain the impact of mental health issues and experiences of family disruption and rejection, on trans young people's decision making about fertility preservation and their reproductive futures.

Poor understandings of reproductive biology was also a factor impacting access to fertility preservation by trans young people. Chen et al. (2017) highlighted the need for young people's greater access to education about fertility, family formation, and identity. Some young people in the study lacked knowledge about basic reproductive biology. For example, one young person believed that pregnancy could occur through using their bone marrow. A trans adolescent presumed female at birth in Chiniara et al.'s (2019) research mentioned they would not need fertility preservation because they would have a biological child, 'as [a] male with his own sperm' (p. 743). As with cis young people, trans young people would benefit from targeted and tailored education about reproduction.

Research indicates that trans young people have minimal access to fertility and fertility preservation education and counselling. Studies focusing on trans adults' perspectives and experiences suggest that healthcare professionals generally do not provide enough information about fertility preservation for trans people to make informed decisions, which may contribute to trans young people not undertaking fertility preservation (Auer et al., 2018). Chen et al. (2017) reported most young people in their study had never discussed fertility or family formation with a healthcare provider (79.5%) or with a parent/guardian (64.7%). Of those young people who had spoken to a healthcare provider about gender-affirming hormones (19.2%), only 53.3% reported their healthcare provider discussed the impact of hormones on fertility.

Researching with trans young people: two Australian studies

This chapter is informed by the findings from two Australian research projects conducted by the authors. The first is a current project – '*Being Trans in the Early Years*' – an exploration of trans children's experiences of social gender affirmation and their parents' experiences at that time. This qualitative study included a focus group with parents (n=7) of children who are trans, aged between 7 and 12 years; and two focus groups with their trans children (n=6). The semi-structured focus group with parents asked an initial opening question: 'Tell us about your experiences parenting a trans child?' This raised discussions about early awareness of and approaches to their children's gender diversity; their understandings of gender and gender diversity; children's social gender affirmation; sources of information about being trans in childhood; perceptions of children's future lives; experiences with schooling and healthcare services; and family supports. This focus group lasted approximately 70 minutes. Additionally, two focus groups were conducted with children: one with three younger children – two were trans boys aged 7, and one was non-binary, aged 8; the second focus group was with three older children who were trans girls, one aged 11 and two aged 12. Throughout the discussion the young people were shown a range of images depicting representations of gender and gender diversity found in popular culture, advertising, media, and children's literature. These images were used to initiate discussion about gender, gender expression and gender diversity, experiences of schooling, and perceptions of their future lives. The focus groups with parents and children were recorded and transcribed verbatim and analysed using inductive thematic approaches and Foucauldian discourse analysis.

The second project – *Growing up Queer* (2014) – involved a mixed-methods approach, including a national online survey of LGBTQ young people aged 16–27, which 1032 participants completed. Thirty-eight per cent (38%) identified as gay, 31% lesbian, 22% bisexual females, and 6% bisexual males. Three per cent (3% or 28 participants) were trans, 10 were trans men and 18 trans women. Forty-five participants were genderqueer or gender diverse. The survey included questions about experiences of homophobia, transphobia, and harassment; experiences of coming out to others; experiences related to identity, health, and wellbeing; and use of the internet and other support resources. Any quotes used in the following discussion of this research are from these two projects unless specified as originating elsewhere, with pseudonyms used for participants' names.

Experiences of cisnormative and heteronormative sexuality education in the Growing Up Queer research

Less than 20% of the LGBTQ+ young people in the *Growing Up Queer* research project reported receiving useful information on trans issues, questioning one's gender, gay, or lesbian relationships, and gay or lesbian safe sex from their school. Young LGBTQ+ people pointed out that any information they did receive in schools and from parents was often transphobic and homophobic. A reoccurring theme in the data was participants' critique of the sexuality education embedded in health education curricula across Australian jurisdictions for being too heteronormative and cisnormative. As reported in the survey by one trans young person: 'I would have benefitted from inclusive sex education in school, not cisnormative and heteronormative sex ed'. Formal in-school education did not address sexual and reproductive health needs of gender and sexuality diverse students, or relevant safe sex practices, sexual pleasure, and wellbeing. Another stated in the survey that they would have liked to have had sexuality education in primary school: 'More education in primary school in being transgender and same-sex attracted'.

Study participants identified that the following areas, in order of most addressed to least addressed content, were generally targeted toward cisgender students only: bodily changes during puberty, human reproduction, STIs, and pregnancy. This was followed by fewer young people receiving information about healthy relationships, sexual rights and responsibilities, or agency and decision making. They pointed out that teachers rarely addressed non-heterosexual relationships. Discussions relevant to trans young people were virtually non-existent. A staff member from the LGBTQIA+ young people's support service commented about trans young people's sexuality education knowledge:

> I feel like there's so many issues that – like even when we were talking about sexual health education … It's not until you actually broach it that young people are like, yeah. I didn't learn anything of use to me in school. I feel like they – it's often – they don't even realise that there's that knowledge gap.
>
> *(Staff member 1)*

Many young people sought out information on the internet, through queer media, popular magazines targeting young people, talking with other LGBTQ+ peers, and learning through personal experiences. The internet was the primary source of information on being trans, sexuality, relationships, and sexual health (e.g., safe sex practices). In terms of finding helpful information about trans issues, 43.1% of young people accessed this information via the internet; 16.9% sourced information from the LGBTQ+ community; 15.6% from specific LGBTQ+ support services; and only 2.9% was from school. Similarly, those young people seeking information about their gender gained this information through the internet (43.3%), followed by the LGBTQ+ community (14.2%), then LGBTQ+ support services (13.1%), and in schools (4.3%). Transgender young people had mixed experiences regarding the usefulness of the internet for relevant information. Some found their searches helpful – others were less enthusiastic. This was reiterated in an interview with another staff member from the LGBTQIA+ young people's support service:

> there's a lot of stuff that they just wouldn't get information about from anywhere … Like, 'I want a transition, I'm going to search for people who have transitioned – had this surgery or whatever and find out their experience'. Trans young people want to search for specific things.
>
> *(Staff member 2)*

In the survey, a trans young person reported that their experiences of searching the internet for relevant information were sometimes far from positive:

> I still question my gender frequently and went through about three years, seriously reviewing who I am/who I was. I mainly used government websites to find out about FtM [female to male] transitions as well as watching YouTube to learn about others and watch the vlog diaries of women who had transitioned to male bodies. I still question my gender and sometimes it triggers my depression again, but after searching myself and the internet I don't believe I'll ever be fully comfortable in the body of a female or male.

Both of our studies highlighted the importance of the internet to young people seeking information about questioning their gender, relationships, and sexual health (Byron, et al., 2017). This searching for some started early in life. However, as relayed by young people, the internet does not always provide the most positive learning environment and nor does it replace the need for off-line discussions with knowledgeable educators. It was also acknowledged that not all young people have access to the internet for various reasons, so alternative sources of information are required.

Trans children and sexuality education: parents' perspectives from the Being Trans in the Early Years project

The parents of trans children in the *Being Trans in the Early Years* project raised concerns about talking to their children about sexuality education. Parents perceived that the discussions they needed to have with their children about puberty and sexuality were different and sometimes more challenging than those facing parents with cisgender children. Parents identified that resources about sexuality education commonly available to parents are inherently focused on cisgender and heterosexual relationships and reproduction. Parents of trans children had to tailor their discussions to the specific needs of their children, with limited access to resources written for transgender young people, as one mother commented:

> When we have to give puberty talks, sex education talks, it's not us picking up a 'Where did I come from' or 'What's happening', we have to tailor things … So there's just probably the same amount of concerns and issues other parents go through, just different concerns and issues.

Parents commented that their children often experience anxiety about attending sexuality education classes at primary school, which are usually separated into binary gender and have minimal benefits for trans young people. Both parents and their trans children considered sexuality education a waste of time. Some indicated that their children are taken out of these classes and given other tasks to complete during these sessions. Apart from being segregated from other children, they also miss out on accessing any relevant sexuality education. Addressing concerns about their child's safety and privacy during school camps or school swimming were also of importance, as raised by a mother, 'We have different concerns like what's going to happen when they go to camp, what's going to happen when they're doing school swimming'. Such issues become significant learning experiences encountered for many of these parents, who often rely on and learn from each other.

Some parents were strong advocates for inclusive sexuality education in their children's schools. They pointed out that schools often believe that they offer children inclusive sexuality education if they address family diversity: 'They think they're inclusive because they talk about people having two mummies and two daddies, but actually it's not inclusive of them' (mother). For the parents in this study, inclusive sexuality education addressing gender and sexuality diversity was considered crucial for not just meeting the needs of trans and sexuality diverse young people, but for *all* young people.

Being Trans in the Early Years project: sexuality education and young trans children (aged 7–8)

Children often engage in play focused on their fantasies of future relationships, largely informed by what they see in their own families and through media. Cis-heteronormative discourses underpin children's play with narratives of marriage, family, mothers and fathers, having babies, and caring for children, represented through children's perspectives of their gendered future lives. All these socio-cultural 'life-stage' milestones, perpetuated through families, media, and education, are generally unquestioned in the early years and viewed as rites of passage to becoming adults; and are mimetically incorporated into children's everyday imaginary worlds (Robinson & Davies, 2015). In the focus groups, young trans children spoke about how they perceived their future relationships with partners. Unlike research with cisgender children (Robinson & Davies, 2015), all three children did not see themselves getting married and having families of their own. However, one child, who identified as a trans boy, did concede that they might change their mind, but quickly reconfirmed, 'I won't get married'.

Parents reported their young children's early anxiety about issues relevant to sexuality education, pointing out that their children often raised problems they were concerned about in their future, including having children. One mother of a trans boy aged eight reported that their child was anxious about other children discovering he did not have a penis and how he would be able to make babies if he did not have one: '[Most] kids aren't thinking about, "mummy, when I want a baby, how am I going to do that? I don't have a penis, and that's where the babies come from"'. Such questions also provoked anxieties in parents, who found it difficult to know how best to answer these questions from their young children, often commenting that it was something they could talk about at another time in the future, as this mother stated to her child: 'Well, we'll get to that later'. This is not an unusual response for a mother of any eight-year-old who is spontaneously, or otherwise, asked a question about sex or reproduction (Robinson, Smith, & Davies, 2017). What this clearly demonstrates is that these young children are dealing with complex questions, including about their bodies and reproductive futures, and need answers to satisfy their curiosity and allay their fears and anxieties.

In relation to all of the young people in the *Being Trans in the Early Years* study, parents reported that their children were generally much more knowledgeable about sexuality education than many of their cisgender peers. The question raised by the eight-year-old trans boy above, shows a level of knowledge about reproduction that is not so common amongst young people of that age, regardless of gender – that is, the penis has a key function in making babies. However, the level of knowledge and understanding that young people have about reproductive biology can vary considerably as discussed previously.

Being Trans in the Early Years project: Trans young people's perspectives of their reproductive futures (ages 11–12)

Understandings of fertility and awareness of fertility preservation options are core to sexuality education relevant to young trans people. In stark contrast to the younger trans children, all three trans girls aged 11–12 years considered having children of their own as core to their future lives. It was an issue that they had all considered. They were well-informed about fertility and fertility preservation, primarily from the counsellors at the gender clinic. For one young person, having a child was a strong wish; she stated, 'I'm dying to have kids. I would absolutely do anything'. This young person wanted to experience carrying a child and giving birth and placed much faith in future scientific reproductive technologies to allow her to carry and bear children. She reported that she would advocate for this in her life: 'I will do whatever I can … I'm going to get involved and I'm going to try and make this happen'.

The 11-year-old girl was still uncertain about having a gonadal biopsy or freezing her gametes. Choosing to freeze their gametes was a decision that weighed heavily on all these young people. The discourse of having a child in the 'natural' or 'normal' way was strong amongst these young people, and feeling this embodiment was especially important. They all spoke about being angered by the comments made by their cisgender young women peers that being a trans girl had some advantages, such as not menstruating:

> 'I'm so sick of girls, non-trans, like, "Oh, your so lucky you don't have to get periods". You're so lucky you don't have a needle jammed in your bum. You're lucky you don't have to have surgery. You're lucky you can have kids'.

One of the 12-year-old trans girls had already decided to freeze their gametes and had had a gonadal biopsy to extract their sperm for future use. The second 12-year-old, just prior to the focus group, had just started the process of fertility preservation and had a recent biopsy. These young people had supported each other through the process, learning what it involved and discussing their concerns with each other. The young person who had most recently started this process commented that their choice was primarily due to their mother's wishes: 'I only had the biopsy because my mum is making me … but yeah I want to do it'. However, there was an acknowledgement that she might regret not having the option of a biological child in the future: 'The reason why I did it is because I don't want to live with – what if I didn't?'

All three young people were also knowledgeable about other options regarding family formation. IVF, egg donation, surrogacy, and adoption were all identified as potential options. For all three participants, adoption was a good option, similar to other research with trans young people (Chen et al. 2017; Nehata et al. 2017), especially if they chose not to have genetically related children, or if that process failed for any reason. Although these young people were aware of many of the legal barriers trans people face, they were less aware of the issues encountered by trans people and adoption, especially in Australia.

In Australia, public health insurance does not cover fertility preservation for trans people, as it is not considered a 'medically necessary' procedure, making it financially prohibitive for many (Smith, Sundstrom, & Delay, 2020; Riggs & Bartholomaeus, 2020). However, research has highlighted the importance of trans young people's access to on-going holistic sexuality education, including reproduction, fertility, and fertility preservation counselling early, before beginning gender-affirming hormone treatment in order to make informed decisions about their futures. There are still uncertainties about the potential impact that long-term exposure to gender-affirming hormones may have on fertility and reproductive functioning (Chen et al., 2017; Knudson & De Sutter, 2017; Brik et al., 2018; Chiniara et al., 2019; Riggs & Bartholomaeus, 2020; Davies, Elder, Riggs, & Robinson, 2021). Lai et al. (2020) argue that there is a lack of in-depth guidance for clinicians and counsellors on trans young people and fertility, including in the WPATH Standards of Care Version 7 developed by the World Professional Association for Transgender Health (WPATH). Lai et al. argue that fertility counselling and fertility preservation for trans young people can be challenging; and that healthcare providers and systems may not be meeting the needs of young trans people.

Socio-cultural barriers to young people's access to holistic sexuality education relevant to their lives

Young people in our research were clearly addressing issues in their early lives that are often viewed as inappropriate by some adults, sometimes even by their supportive parents. Socio-cultural barriers associated with childhood impact the regulation of the content and quality of sexuality education to which children and young people have access in their schooling, at home, and in health settings. The discourse of childhood innocence has been foundational to many adults' perceptions that children require protection, for as long as possible, from what are considered 'adults-only' issues, viewed to be dangerous and risky for children and young people — sexuality education, especially LGBTQ issues, has been very much at the forefront of these concerns (Robinson, 2013; Robinson, Smith & Davies, 2017). The discourse of childhood innocence fosters perceptions about children as 'too young' to emotionally and cognitively understand concepts included in sexuality education, with some adults believing that this information is developmentally inappropriate and therefore harmful for children. However, research shows that gender and sexuality development starts early in life and children are building understandings of 'special' relationships, romantic love, intimacy, forming families, and having children, despite some adult's perceptions that these issues are irrelevant to their lives (Blaise, 2010; Renold, 2005;

Robinson, 2013; Robinson & Davies, 2015). Research (Riley et al., 2011; Grant et al., 2011) shows that children are expressing their gender, including gender diversity, by the age of three – also demonstrated in our research with trans children and young people.

Adolescence is often considered a time of risk-taking and challenging boundaries, and a time of emotional and physical changes. It is during this time that young people are often focused on their gender and sexuality. There is a prevailing myth that sexuality education encourages young people to become sexually active too early. However, research has shown that good-quality, holistic sexuality education does not lead to early sexual debut; in fact, it can lead to young people having their first sexual encounters later and involve more responsible sexual behaviour (European Expert Group on Sexuality Education, 2016; UNESCO 2009; Van Keulen et al., 2015). Adolescents are commonly making decisions about their sexual and reproductive lives which may have lifelong consequences. Adolescents, like adults, make decisions in their own best interests with the information they have available and should be supported to do this with agency. They have a right to be informed about gender and sex, fertility and sexuality, so the decisions they make are informed decisions (Pang et al., 2021).

Conclusion

Sexuality education in schools, which is framed within heteronormative cisgender discourses, does not meet the needs of young trans people, or those who are sexuality diverse, or those young people who are questioning their gender and/or sexuality. Sexuality education can perpetuate transphobic and homophobic perspectives of transgender people, through rendering them invisible, or through misinformation. As such, sexuality education in schools continues to be irrelevant and often anxiety provoking for trans young people. This becomes even more concerning as not all trans young people have access to evidence-based sexuality education from parents, other family members, healthcare professionals, or from community services. The internet is an important source of information for young people, but it can be difficult to navigate vast amounts of information, and can be an alienating and isolating experience for some young people.

Research that includes young people's perspectives on fertility and fertility preservation raise some important concerns for reconceptualising sexuality education for trans children and young people, and needs to begin early in life. Sexuality education is essential for providing trans young people with the evidence-based information they require to make informed decisions about sex, sexuality, relationships, formation of future families, fertility, and reproductive futures (Riggs & Bartholomaeus, 2020). It is also crucial that trans children, adolescents, and their families have enough information to be able to discuss these issues and to answer questions they may have related to sexuality education. Good quality relevant sexuality education is foundational to all young people becoming healthily informed, resilient, competent, and respectful sexual citizens.

References

Auer, M. K., Fuss, J. O., Nieder, T., Briken, P., Biedermann, S. V., Stalla, G. K., Beckmann, M. W., & Hildebrandt, T. (2018). Desire to have children among transgender people in Germany: A cross-sectional multi-center study. *Journal of Sexual Medicine*, 15(5), 757–767.

Bartholomaeus, C., & Riggs, D. W. (2017) *Transgender people and education*. New York: Palgrave Macmillan.

Blaise, M. (2010). Kiss and tell: gendered narratives and childhood sexuality. *Australasian Journal of Early Childhood*, 35(1), 1–9.

Brik, T., Vrouenraets, L. J. J. J., Schagen, S. E. E., Meissner, A., de Vries, M. C., & Hannema, S. E. (2018). Use of fertility preservation among a cohort of transgirls in the Netherlands. *Society for Adolescent Health and Medicine*, 64(5), 589–593.

Byron, P., Rasmussen, S., Wright Toussaint, D., Lobo, R., Robinson, K. H., & Paradise, B. (2017). *'You learn from each other': LGBTIQ young people's mental health help-seeking and the RAD Australia online directory*. Western Sydney University and Young and Well Cooperative Research Centre, Sydney. Retrieved from http://handle.westernsydney.edu.au:8081/1959.7/uws:38815

Chen, D., Matson, M., Macapagal, K., Johnson, E. K., Rosoklija, I., Finlayson, C., Fisher, C. B., & Mustanski, B. (2017). Attitudes toward fertility and reproductive health among transgender and gender-nonconforming adolescents. *Journal of Adolescent Health*, 63(1), 62–68.

Chiniara, L. N., Viner, C., Palmert, M., Bonifacio, H. (2019). Perspectives on fertility preservation and parenthood among transgender youth and their parents, *Archives of Disease in Childhood*, 104, 739–744.

Davies, C. Elder, C. V., Riggs, D. W., & Robinson, K. H. (2021). The importance of informed fertility counselling for trans young people. *The Lancet Child and Adolescent Health*, correspondence, 5(9), e36–e37.

European Expert Group on Sexuality Education (2016). Sexuality education – what is it? *Sex Education: Sexuality, Society and Learning*, 16(4), 27–431.

Ferfolja, T., & Ullman, J. (2021). *Gender and sexuality diversity in a culture of limitation*. London: Routledge.

Grant, J. M., Mottet, L. A., Tanis, J., Harrison, J., Herman, J. L., Keisling, M. (2011). *Injustice at every turn: A report of the National Transgender Discrimination Survey*. Washington, DC: National Center for Transgender Equality and National Gay and Lesbian Task Force.

Hillier, L., Jones, T., Monagle, M., Overton, N., Gahan, L., Blackman, J., & Mitchell. A. (2010). *Writing themselves in 3: The third national study on the sexual health and wellbeing of same-sex attracted and gender questioning young people*. Melbourne: Australian Research Centre in Sex, Health and Society, La Trobe University.

Kosciw, J. G., Clark, C. M., Truong, N. L., & Zongrone, A. D. (2020). *The 2019 National School Climate Survey: The experiences of lesbian, gay, bisexual, transgender, and queer youth in our nation's schools*. New York: GLSEN.

Knudson, G., & De Sutter, P. (2017) Fertility options in transgender and gender diverse adolescents. Nordic Federation of Societies of Obstetrics and Gynecology, *Acta Obstetricia at Gynecologica Scandinavica*, 96, 1269–1272.

Lai, T., Davies, C., Robinson, K. H., Feldman, D., Elder, C., Cooper, C., Pang, K. C., McDougall, R. (2021). Effective fertility counselling for transgender adolescents: a qualitative study of clinician attitudes and practices, *British Medical Journal Open*, 11(5), e043237.

Lai, T. C., McDougall, R., Feldman, D., Elder, C., & Pang, K. (2020). Fertility counseling for transgender adolescents: A review. *Journal of Adolescent Health*, 66, 658–665.

Lawlis, S. M., Donkin, H. R., Bates, J. R., Britto, M. T., & Conard, L. A. E. (2017). Health concerns of transgender and gender nonconforming youth and their parents upon presentation to a transgender clinic. *Journal of Adolescent Health, 61*, 642–648.

Lopez, G. (2017). Trump just made it official: Transgender students no longer have an ally in the White House. *Vox*, February 22. Retrieved April 23, 2022 from www.vox.com/identities/2017/2/22/14683572/trump-transgender-schools-guidance

McGowan, M. (2022). 'Targeted discrimination': NSW government rejects Mark Latham's trans bill. *The Guardian*, Wednesday, March 16. Retrieved April 23, 2022 from www.theguardian.com/australia-news/2022/mar/16/targeted-discrimination-nsw-government-rejects-mark-lathams-trans-bill

Nehata, L., Tishelman, A.C., Caltabellotta, B.A., Quinn, G.P. (2017) Low fertility preservation utilization among transgender youth. *Journal of Adolescent Health, 61*, 40–44.

New South Wales Department of Education (2021). *Controversial issues in schools*. New South Wales Department of Education, Sydney, Australia. Retrieved May 14, 2022 from https://education.nsw.gov.au/policy-library/policies/pd-2002-0045#:~:text=Policy%20statement,-The%20study%20of&text=Controversial%20issues%20are%20managed%20in,interest%20of%20any%20particular%20group

Owen, G. (2017). Adolescence, trans phenomena, and the politics of sexuality education. In L. Allen & M. Rasmussen (Eds.), *The Palgrave handbook of sexuality education* (pp. 555–570). London: Palgrave Macmillan.

Pang, K. C., Giordano, S., Sood, N., & Skinner, S. R. (2021). Regret, informed decision making, and respect for autonomy of trans young people. *The Lancet, Child & Adolescent Health*, Correspondence, *5*(9), E34–E35.

Pang, K. C., Peri, A. J. S., Chung, H. E., Telfer, M., Elder, C. V., Grover, S., & Jayasinghe, Y. (2020). Rates of fertility preservation use among transgender adolescents. *JAMA Pediatrics, 174*, 890–891.

Renold, E. (2005). *Girls, boys, and junior sexualities: Exploring children's gender and sexual relationships in the primary school*. London: Routledge Falmer.

Riggs, D. W. (2013). Heteronormativity in online information about sex: A South Australian case study. *Contemporary Issues in Early Childhood, 14*(1), 72–80.

Riggs, D. W., & Bartholomaeus, C. (2020). Towards trans reproductive justice: A qualitative analysis of views on fertility preservation for Australian transgender and non-binary people. *Journal of Social Issues, 76*(2), 314–337.

Riggs, D. W., & Bartholomaeus, C. (2018). Transgender young people's narratives of intimacy and sexual health: Implications for sexuality education. *Sex Education, 18*, 376–390.

Riley, E. A., Sitharthan, G., Clemson, L., & Diamond, M. (2011). The needs of gender-variant children and their parents: A parent survey. *International Journal of Sexual Health, 23*(3), 181–195.

Robinson, K. H. (2022). Children's sexual citizenship. In N. Fischer, L. Westbrook & S. Seidman (Eds.), *Introducing the new sexualities studies* (4th ed., pp. 730–738). New York: Routledge.

Robinson, K. H. (2012). Difficult citizenship: The precarious relationships between childhood, sexuality and access to knowledge. *Sexualities, 15*(3/4), 257–276.

Robinson, K. H. (2013) *Innocence, knowledge and the construction of childhood: The contradictory nature of sexuality and censorship in children's contemporary lives*. London: Routledge.

Robinson, K. H., & Davies, C. (2017). Sexuality education in early childhood. In L. Allen & M. Rasmussen (Eds.), *Handbook of sexuality education*. London: Palgrave.

Robinson, K. H., Smith, E., & Davies, C. (2017. Responsibilities, tensions and ways forward: Parents' perspectives on children's sexuality education. *Sex Education, 17*(3), 333–347.

Robinson, K. H., & Davies, C. (2015). Children's gendered and sexual cultures: Desiring and regulating recognition through life markers of marriage, love and relationships. In E. Renold, J. Ringrose & D.R. Egan (Eds.), *Children, Sexuality & Sexualization*. London: Palgrave.

Robinson, K. H., & Davies, C. (2008) Docile bodies and heteronormative moral subjects: Constructing the child and sexual knowledge in schools, *Sexuality and Culture*, 12(4), 221–239.

Shannon, B. (2022). *Sex(uality) education for trans and gender diverse youth in Australia*. London: Palgrave Macmillan.

Smith, E., Jones, T., Ward, R., Dixon, J., Mitchell, A., & Hillier, L. (2014). *From blues to rainbows: Mental health and wellbeing of gender diverse and transgender young people in Australia*. Melbourne: The Australian Research Centre in Sex, Health, and Society.

Smith, E., Sundstrom, B., & Delay, C. (2020). Listening to women: Understanding and challenging systems of power to achieve reproductive justice in South Carolina. *Journal of Social Issues*, 76(2), 363–390.

Strang, J. F., Jarin, J., Call, D., Clark, B., Wallace, L., Anthony, L. G., Kenworthy, L., & Gomez-Lobo, V. (2018). Transgender youth fertility attitudes questionnaire: Measure development in nonautistic and autistic transgender youth and their parents. *Journal of Adolescent Health*, 62(2), 128–135.

Terence Higgins Trust. (2019). New sex education guidance a step forward but LGBT inclusion must be mandatory. Press Release, 25th February. Retrieved April 23, 2022 from www.tht.org.uk/news/new-sex-education-guidance-step-forward-lgbt-inclusion-must-be-mandatory

UNESCO. (2018). *International technical guidance on sexuality education: An evidence-informed approach*. UNESCO: France. Retrieved May 14, 2022 from https://cdn.who.int/media/docs/default-source/reproductive-health/sexual-health/international-technical-guidance-on-sexuality-education.pdf?sfvrsn=10113efc_29&download=true

Van Keulen, H. M., Hofstetter, H., Peters, L. W. H., Meijer, S., Schutte, L., & Van Empelen, P. (2015). *Effectiveness of the Long Live Love 4 Program for 13- and 14-year-old secondary school students in the Netherlands: A quasi-experimental design*. Delft: Organization for Applied Scientific Research (TNO).

Walton-Betancourth, S., Monti, E., Adu-Gyamfi, K., Roberts, A., Clarkson, K., Ward, S., & Butler, G. (2018). Fertility preservation for transgender adolescents: The parent's view. *Endocrine Abstracts*, 58, P030.

WHO Regional Office for Europe and BZgA. (2010). *Standards for sexuality education in Europe: A framework for policy makers, education and health authorities and specialists*. Köln: BZgA.

7

ERASURE OF IDENTITY OR GENDER EUPHORIA

The impact of cancer on trans embodiment

*Jane M. Ussher, Rosalie Power, Kimberley Allison,
Samantha Sperring, Chloe Parton, Janette Perz,
Cristyn Davies, Alexandra J. Hawkey, Kerry H. Robinson,
Martha Hickey, Antoinette Anazodo, Colin Ellis and
Teddy Cook*

Introduction

There is a pressing need for attention to be paid to the cancer survivorship and cancer caring experiences of transgender (trans, binary, and non-binary) people, in order to inform practice and policy, and the development of culturally safe cancer information and care (Pratt-Chapman, Alpert, & Castillo, 2021; Ussher, Perz et al., 2022). Research in the emerging area of lesbian, gay, bisexual, trans, queer, and intersex (LGBTQI) cancer survivorship largely tends to assume cisgender embodiment, identity, and expression (Taylor & Bryson, 2016), with few trans people included in study samples (Pratt-Chapman et al., 2021). A small minority of studies focus on survivorship outcomes (Boehmer, Gereige, Winter, Ozonoff, & Scout, 2020) and healthcare experiences (Alpert et al., 2021; Kerr, Fisher, & Jones, 2020; Squires, Bilash, Kamen, & Garland, 2022; Taylor & Bryson, 2016), drawing on the experiences of small samples of trans individuals.

Minimal attention has been paid to the impact of cancer on trans identity and embodiment, and the ways in which trans people negotiate these aspects of experience in the context of cancer and cancer care. By embodiment we mean the experience of living in, perceiving, and experiencing the world from the location of our gendered bodies and the ways in which our social environments "enter into and become entangled with our bodies" (Tolman, Bowman, & Fahs, 2014, p. 761). This chapter will review current knowledge about experiences of identity and embodiment for trans people with cancer and trans cancer carers, including their interactions with healthcare professionals (HCPs), drawing on existing literature, as well as the findings of our recently completed Out with Cancer Study (Power, Ussher et al., 2022; Ussher, Allison, Perz, Power, & The Out with Cancer Study Team, 2022; Ussher, Perz et al., 2022; Ussher, Power et al., 2022). Before outlining the study methodology, we begin by examining existing literature on cancer risk factors which may be unique for trans people.

DOI: 10.4324/9781003138310-7

Cancer risk, screening, and diagnosis: are trans people at higher risk for cancer?

Research on cancer in trans communities has primarily focused on epidemiology, aetiology, and biomedical aspects of cancer treatment (Watters, Harsh, & Corbett, 2015). Data on the prevalence of cancer amongst trans populations is limited, partly due to the non-collection of information about gender and sexuality diversity in cancer registries and decentralisation of trans healthcare (Brown & Jones, 2015). However, US data suggests a higher prevalence of cancer amongst trans men, relative to cis men, while the prevalence amongst trans women and non-binary people appears comparable to that amongst cis men and women (Boehmer et al., 2020). Reasons for the elevated risk of cancer are unclear, but may include higher rates of known cancer risks amongst trans populations, such as HPV and HIV infection, smoking and alcohol use, and medical comorbidities (Boehmer et al., 2020; Grant, Mottet, & Tanis, 2011). Increased risk of HPV infection, and by extension some cancers, has also been associated with vaginoplasty (Puechl, Russell, & Gray, 2019). There have also been suggestions that exogenous hormone use as part of gender affirmation may be a risk factor (Kerr, Fisher, & Jones, 2019). In the largest cohort of trans people in Europe, trans women on gender affirmation hormone therapy (GAHT) were observed to have a higher risk of breast cancer than cis men, but a lower risk compared with cis women (Jackson, Nambiar, O'Callaghan, & Berner, 2022). Higher rates of positive cervical pap tests have been reported in trans men, compared to cisgender women (Peitzmeier, Reisner, Harigopal, & Potter, 2014). However, larger, longer-term studies suggest exogenous hormones may not be a cancer risk factor for trans people (Brown & Jones, 2015; Taylor & Bryson, 2016), and there is agreement on the pressing need for longitudinal research in this sphere (Jackson, et al., 2022).

Trans populations may experience significant complications in the cancer diagnostic process as a result of socioeconomic issues, including higher rates of poverty, lower rates of health insurance (Grant et al., 2011), and previous negative experiences with healthcare (Kerr et al., 2020). Trans people report low rates of cancer screening (Oladeru et al., 2022), particularly for gendered cancers, such as breast, cervical, and prostate cancer, due to previous negative experiences during screening, reluctance to attend gendered health services, and dysphoria associated with screening (Connolly, Hughes, & Berner, 2020). This is compounded by, and a pervasive "silence" and "invisibility" around trans people in cancer awareness campaigns (Braun et al., 2017; Deebel et al., 2017). Trans people may be excluded from screening reminders or invitations to screen for relevant gendered cancers because of the ways their gender is listed in medical records (Connolly et al., 2020). These delays and avoidance of care may lead to cancers remaining undetected or being diagnosed at a later stage, and in combination with behavioural risk factors and medical comorbidities (Boehmer et al., 2020; Grant et al., 2011), may contribute to poorer outcomes amongst trans people with cancer.

Impact of cancer on trans identity and embodiment: the Out with Cancer Study

For trans people diagnosed with cancer, both the symptoms of cancer and the cancer treatment may affect gender identity, embodiment and processes of gender affirmation. In the Out with Cancer Study, we found significantly higher levels of distress in trans participants in comparison to the cis participants, with distress associated with impact of cancer on trans identity (Ussher, Allison, et al., 2022). In qualitative analysis we identified heightened gender dysphoria and interrupted gender affirmation as the primary negative impacts of cancer on identity. However, for some trans individuals, cancer interventions had a positive impact, reflected in gender euphoria – comfort or joy in ones gender – and facilitation of gender affirmation, the interpersonal, interactive process whereby trans individuals receive social recognition and support for their gender identity and expression (Nuttbrock et al., 2009). Interactions with HCPs had the potential to exacerbate or ameliorate the negative impact of cancer on trans identity and embodiment.

Before elaborating upon these findings, we will briefly describe the methodology of the Out with Cancer study. We examined cancer survivorship and care experiences of 430 LGBTQI cancer patients and survivors and 130 carers, including 63 patients and 23 carers who identified as trans, using a combination of survey, interviews, and photovoice (Ussher, Allison, et al., 2022; Ussher, Power, et al., 2022). We also examined the perspectives of 357 healthcare professionals (HCPs) on LGBTQI cancer care, including working with trans people (Ussher Perz et al., 2022). Full details of the methodology and study sample are provided elsewhere (Ussher, Allison, et al., 2022; Ussher, Power, et al., 2022). In this chapter, we draw on the accounts of the 86 trans cancer survivors (n=63) and carers (n=23), who represented a broad range of cancer types (including breast, prostate, uterine, colorectal, head and neck, leukaemia, melanoma, other) and age groups (mean age 42, range 17–72 years), with 18 identifying as trans women, 10 as trans men and 53 as non-binary, genderfluid, or genderqueer. The majority (90.0%) were Caucasian, identifying as lesbian, gay, or homosexual (23.8%), bisexual (27.7%), queer (25.4%), or multiple sexual identities (14.3%), with a minority identifying as heterosexual (9.5%). The majority lived in Australia (57%) or the United States (20.6%), in an urban (48.4%), regional (41.9%), or rural (9.7%) location. Seventeen (33%) of the trans participants reported an intersex variation (14 cancer survivors, 3 carers), the majority of whom had experienced medical intervention to prevent cancer. Following principles of integrated knowledge translation (iKT) (Graham et al., 2006), LGBTQI cancer survivors – including individuals who identified as trans, cancer HCPs and representatives from LGBTQI health and cancer support organisations were involved in all stages of the project. The project adopts an intersectional theoretical framework, which acknowledges that individuals inhabit multiple interconnected social identity categories, such as gender, sexuality, cultural background, and age (Crenshaw, 1991), and that these identity categories are embedded in systems of social stratification, associated with inequality or power (Hawkey & Ussher, 2022; Marecek, 2016; Warner, 2008).

"Terrible gender dysphoria": cancer treatment erases gender affirmation

Trans populations report significantly higher rates of depression, anxiety, and suicidal ideation than cis populations, associated with gender dysphoria and minority
stress (Clements-Nolle, Marx, & Katz, 2006; James et al., 2016). Gender dysphoria is a complex and nuanced experience of suffering, in response to internal and
external stimuli which produce a disconnection between one's internal understanding of self and the external presentation of self (Austin, Papciak, & Lovins, 2022).
Cancer and cancer treatment impacts may potentially heighten gender dysphoria,
with distress associated with embodied change following cancer most notable for
those with cancers of highly gendered body parts, such as breasts or reproductive
organs. For example, cancer of the uterus has been constructed through gendered
discourses such as a "woman's cancer", aligning internal organs with a person's
gender identity. These dominant discourses may be discordant with trans masculine
or non-binary identities, resulting in distress. As a trans man diagnosed with uterine
cancer told us:

> The type of cancer I have had which relates to my sex assigned at birth can
> be distressing and is hard to cope with and brings about a lot of dysphoria. It's
> more having a stupid cancer associated with my organs I don't want and were
> taken out but still I have to deal with when I just want to forget they even
> existed and don't want to think about that stuff ever.
>
> *(Trans man, queer, age 34, uterine)*

Similar experiences of gender dysphoria for trans men have been reported in relation to cervical cancer screening, with the need "to focus on an essentially female
part" during a pap test described as "incredibly upsetting" (Johnson, Nemeth,
Mueller, Eliason, & Stuart, 2016).

Some cancers are treated using hormone therapies, while others are
hormone-sensitive, in both cases interacting with hormones used as part of gender affirmation. Cancer treatment decisions may thus have significant and enduring impacts on trans cancer survivors' gender identity and expression (Taylor &
Bryson, 2016). For example, a trans lesbian woman with melanoma, aged 40,
told us "it [diagnosis] came so soon after I began my transition and I was happy
for the first time in my life and then in the blink of an eye, that brief feeling
of elation was cut short. That sucked". The physical impact of hormones used
during fertility preservation can also have a material and psychological impact on
experiences of gendered embodiment. A trans carer reported experiencing "cata-
strophic depression" and "terrible gender dysphoria" as a result of his engagement
in fertility preservation treatment some years ago, to preserve an embryo before
his partner received cancer treatment. He told us "when I was given steroids to
provoke ovulation, I attempted suicide because of how fucked up my trans brain
responded to even more oestrogen" (trans man, queer, age 53, carer of partner
with thyroid cancer).

Mastectomy following breast cancer may be perceived to "erase" an individual's experience and expression of gender nonconformity (Taylor & Bryson, 2016), or affect the self-perceived femininity of a trans woman. As an Out with Cancer Study participant told us:

> As a trans woman, I was very pleased that my body developed breasts naturally at around age 45. I was not taking hormones. I wanted an orchidectomy, but when I contacted specialists, I was advised that due to very high cancer risk due to family history, that I had to have a bilateral mastectomy. In hindsight, I wish that I hadn't had the mastectomy. Having natural breasts was a big part of my female identity.
>
> *(Trans woman, unsure sexuality, 56, intervention to reduce cancer risk)*

Other bodily changes such as treatment-related hair loss, lymphedema, weight gain or loss, and changes to sexual functioning, may impact embodied experience. For example, a trans man told us of the trauma of losing his facial hair during chemotherapy, which resulted in him being "misgendered as a woman":

> There was no support, recognition or understanding of the impact of losing the beard hair being a transman. I had to sit across from women getting fussed over and getting head cool pack things to try to stop their hair loss. There was no recognition or help for my loss, so linked to my identity.
>
> *(Trans man, gay, age 55, multiple)*

Weight changes can also lead to misgendering and dysphoria. A trans man with ovarian cancer explained how his masculinity was challenged by treatment-related weight gain: "the lymphedema causes me gender dysphoria because it feminizes my abdomen/hips" (age 47, heterosexual). Another participant contrasted the feminising impact of lymphedema with masculinising "top surgery":

> If top surgery is more like masc-presenting with lymphedema is like ultra-femme because you get swollen and you get curvy and you get lumps in different areas. And you, like, all of the lymphedema stuff is like ultra-femme, it's like pink or tan.
>
> *(Non-binary, queer, 37, multiple)*

A number of trans intersex participants reported feelings of "shame" associated with the impact of medical intervention to prevent cancer on the sexual body. A participant who described having had "gonadectomy at age 4" told us "it really does impact on my sexual wellbeing and intimacy, because of scar tissue, because of shame and because I always wonder what it would be like had I not had the gonadectomy so young" (non-binary, lesbian, intersex, 25). Others talked about the impact of hormonal treatments on sexual functioning. For example, a non-binary queer breast cancer survivor, age 49 said that "tamoxifen drew me into menopause and I wasn't feeling very sexual … I mourn that part … it wasn't for me about how I looked it was just about how I feel internally". Cancer related embodied changes may be complicated by gender-affirming medical procedures, with an impact on gendered and sexual embodiment. Urinary incontinence following vaginoplasty can be exacerbated by cancer treatment, and may also impact on bowel incontinence (Jiang, Gallagher, Burchill, Berli, & Dugi, 2019). Dilation of the neovaginal canal to prevent stenosis may also be impacted by vaginal dryness following cancer surgery (Ingham, Lee, MacDermed, & Olumi, 2018). In combination, this suggests that the intersection of cancer treatment and gender affirmation, at a material, discursive, and intrapsychic level, needs to be taken into account by HCPs and those providing health information for trans people with cancer.

"I put it on hold": cancer caring interrupts gender affirmation

Caring for a person with cancer can also interrupt the process of gender affirmation. For example, a 26-year-old queer cis woman with lymphoma, whose partner was a trans woman, told us that cancer delayed both of their processes of "coming out" to family, saying "I don't want to rock the boat right now because I don't think my parents are going to be very accepting. I don't want to have to deal with that on top of cancer". For others, caring took up all of their emotional energy, and "dealing with" gender affirmation was "put on hold" or "put to the side", because "it just wasn't something that either of us were able to even consider looking at and talking about … it was very much a focus on you just had to survive" (non-binary, queer, age 38, caring for partner with breast cancer). This participant also reported "immense guilt regarding wanting top surgery because my partner has had a mastectomy to save her life due to the cancer". Gender affirmation and coming out in relation to sexuality were often interconnected. A 20-year-old bisexual non-binary person caring for their father with brain cancer told us:

> I was still discovering my sexuality when I was a carer and felt like I didn't have the emotional energy to deal with it so tried to think about it as little as possible. I was not out when I was caring.

Concealing trans identity and passing as cis was positioned as a necessary part of the caring role by several participants in the Out with Cancer Study. This is a common strategy of self-protection for trans people (Levitt & Ippolito, 2014); however, the strategy of hiding one's true gender identity can be associated with a diminished sense of self and magnified dysphoria (Cole, Denny, Eyler, & Samons, 2002). For example, a 38-year-old queer non-binary person caring for their grandmother with bowel cancer said:

> While I was a carer that role came before my own needs as non-binary; I stopped taking hormones and presented as more feminine. As a carer I was less open about being non-binary as I did not want it to affect me or my grandmother's needs.

This had negative intrapsychic consequences, as having "to feel that I had to pretend to be someone else was upsetting and stressful". It also had consequences in terms of isolation and support, as they continued: "I felt more isolated from the LGBTIQ+ community while I was a carer. I did not feel supported and also stopped interacting with this part of the community". These accounts demonstrate the negative impact of gender affirmation being "put aside" because of caring, serving to compound the many other factors associated with distress for cancer carers (Perz, Ussher, Butow, & Wain, 2011), creating greater vulnerability for trans carers.

"I'm more connected with my body": cancer increases gender euphoria

Reports of a negative impact of cancer on trans identity were not universal in the Out with Cancer Study. Cancer diagnosis can result in ambivalent feelings around identity for some trans people. For example, for trans men with reproductive cancers, relief at the absence of menstruation may be tempered by being diagnosed with a "woman's cancer". As a participant told us "the symptoms both brought me relief [lack of periods] and torment, years of being misdiagnosed, having constant focus on my 'womanhood', which had a huge impact on me as a transgender man" (trans man, straight, age 38, ovarian). The removal of ovaries was associated with "some grief about the loss of those parts (that) were part of me" for a trans man we interviewed, but he went on say, this "doesn't affect my masculinity" because "there's lots of nuances to being transgender" (straight, 47, ovarian).

For others, cancer treatments can serve to facilitate the process of gender affirmation and increase gender euphoria – positive feelings in response to affirmation of one's body or gender identity, including comfort, confidence, certainty, satisfaction, and joy (Austin et al., 2022). Hormonal cancer treatment can have a positive defeminising effect for trans masculine people, rarely recognised within dominant cis-heteronormative discourses of cancer care (Ussher, Power, et al., 2022). This is exemplified in the account of a 52-year-old trans man with thyroid cancer who said the information from HCPs "that 'we are sorry to say that one possible unpleasant side effect of chemo is that you may …' was very confusing, as all the 'negative' de-feminising side effects caused internal gender euphoria". Removal of the uterus following diagnosis of ovarian cancer can lead to feelings of "relief" and a sense of wholeness, epitomising gender euphoria: "It was like a million bricks flying off of my shoulders when I woke up from surgery. And I didn't have these parts in me anymore. I felt more whole than I had in my entire life" (trans man, straight, age 47, ovarian). In a similar vein, a genderqueer participant in a study by Alpert and colleagues described their loss of ovaries as a "godsend" (Alpert et al., 2021).

Reductions in erectile function and penis size, often accompanied by feminising bodily changes, are common consequences of prostate cancer treatment which have a negative impact on the psychological wellbeing and identity of cis gay and bisexual men, resulting in a sense of "sexual disqualification" (Ussher et al., 2017). For trans people, these same embodied changes can be positive and affirming of identity, as a trans woman taking hormone therapy for prostate cancer told us: "having a shorter and non-erect penis is a positive for me, as is reduced muscle mass and strength and breast sensitivity – at least now I have breasts that are sensitive" (gay, 63). Reduction in testicle size is a further consequence of prostate cancer treatment, which can have positive consequences for trans women.

> Hormone blockers mean that my testicles, well they're very small now, and I don't care if they stay there because I can wear tighter panties and hide everything, Nothing shows, really …. It is good the HRT for being trans-gender and the treatment for cancer is one and the same, which makes me very happy.
>
> *(Trans woman, 63, prostate)*

Several studies have indicated that trans and sexuality diverse patients have begun to embrace the choice to forego breast reconstruction after mastectomy (Brown & McElroy, 2018; Rubin & Tanenbaum, 2011; Wandrey, Qualls, & Mosack, 2016). A bilateral mastectomy is medically similar to gender-affirming "top surgery", which may facilitate an alignment between masculine or non-binary gender identity and embodiment (Taylor & Bryson, 2016). Some trans individuals decide to "go flat" (also known as "flattopping"), as a genderqueer participant from Brown and McElroy's (2018) study explained after making this treatment choice, "I feel like I now have a body that fits me" (p. 411). A number of trans participants in the Out with Cancer Study echoed this sentiment: "I'm more connected with my gender non-conforming identity. Breasts caused me some dysphoria …. clothes fit better now I don't have to hide breasts in them somehow" (non-binary, lesbian, 52, breast); "I knew I wanted to live flat, so in an 'odd' way, cancer allowed me to achieve the flat chest and breastless body I wanted" (non-binary, queer, age 37, multiple cancers). However, it is important to note that the aesthetics, mobility, and recovery resulting from mastectomy without reconstruction often vary greatly to that of top surgery. As a trans participant who was living flat explained:

> [double mastectomy] itself is a very different procedure. They remove every bit of breast tissue … You don't get pecs, you don't get nipples – I don't have nipples. You don't get to have a body that resembles any mainstream body. You just have to take whatever comes out at the other end of that surgery, and for some people that means they have lumpy bits here and there or dog ears or concaved chests, and for other people that means that they get really flat smooth chests; everyone has a different physical response to mastectomy surgery. And for me it's been nothing like top surgery … I still can't reach above my shoulders; I can't reach up high or reach the middle of a table or pick up something from the ground easily … [top surgery] is far more recoverable.
>
> *(Non-binary, queer, 37, breast)*

The outcome of mastectomy without reconstruction for these participants is positioned as unlike top surgery, and *lacking* elements of "mainstream" masculinity. According to Foster (2021), "a mastectomy can be a part of top surgery, but not every top surgery is a full mastectomy".

Assumptions about changes in embodiment for people with cancer, including within healthcare settings, are generally underpinned by dominant discourses of binary gender. The majority of studies indicate that both trans and sexuality diverse cis women face considerable pressure to undergo breast reconstruction after mastectomy, from both survivor organisations and within the medical system (Brown & McElroy, 2018; Rubin & Tanenbaum, 2011). Meanings attached to embodied change are individual and assumptions cannot be made about the impact of cancer treatment for a generic "LGBTQI" population, as is sometimes the case in health information (Pratt-Chapman et al., 2021). This suggests a need for HCPs to be educated about cis-heteronormative assumptions, as well as the availability of gender neutral resources and information regarding treatment options (Sinding, Grassau, & Barnoff, 2007).

"The genie came out of the bottle": cancer facilitates gender affirmation

For some, a cancer diagnosis can facilitate or confirm the decision to engage in gender affirmation. For example, for one Out with Cancer Study participant, being told that they needed a mastectomy "was the moment that the genie came out of the bottle" allowing them acknowledged their true identity as a trans man, because of the "utter relief and awareness they [breasts] so long ago should have been off" (trans man, gay, age 55, multiple cancers). For others, cancer caused them to reflect on what is important in life, and be "more open about being a non-binary trans person" (gender fluid non-binary, queer, pansexual, 32, testicular), or "come to terms with" their trans identity.

> But then when I got diagnosed with cancer, it made me … focus on that a lot more, about … actually, who am I, and how do I want to continue, and … at what point am I going to ignore these parts of myself. So, coming to terms with it's been a recent thing anyway. Or not coming to terms with it, but being vocal about it.
>
> *(Non-binary, gay, 32, leukaemia)*

Partners and other carers can also experience a realisation of their trans identity, or have the confidence to engage in gender affirmation, because of their cancer caring experience. A trans woman told us that her "transition [occurred] through that period" of caring for her partner with breast cancer, following a discussion of "how we would spend our last day. And that led to me confessing to her that I'd rather spend the last day of my life authentically [as a trans woman]" (bisexual, intersex, 59). A non-binary participant told us that they realised the "disconnect" with their body and their "suppressed" feelings about gender affirmation when they witnessed their partner's distress at the loss of her breasts:

> Witnessing her going through that kind of made me realize my disconnect with my own body. … I guess it just kind of like triggered me to actually connect just those feelings I've had for a really long time. You do what you can to suppress anything that's too difficult to talk about. And it just kind of triggered a journey for me to start processing some stuff which I never processed before …. I think in new situations I feel like I can like present who I am now.
>
> *(Non-binary, queer, 32, caring for partner with breast cancer)*

Navigating cis-heteronormative cancer care: interactions with healthcare professionals

"A complete lack of understanding": HCPs negate or pathologise trans embodiment

To practice trans inclusive cancer care, HCPs need to understand the intersection of cancer and trans embodiment (Jackson et al., 2022; Winter et al., 2016). In the Out with Cancer study, reports of HCPs ignoring or denying the impact of cancer treatment on trans embodiment were common. For example, a non-binary prostate cancer survivor told us there was "no alternative offered to radical prostatectomy, no consideration of my transgender status". This had implications for their ability to medically transition, which left them feeling "cheated":

> To be honest if they had been more understanding and listened to me I could have had a bottom transition operation. Rather than being left without any ability [for medical gender affirmation] and no chance of transition due to the extensive damage done.
>
> *(Non-binary gender fluid, 68, prostate and pancreatic)*

A breast cancer survivor who told "a team of female doctors" that they would "rather have [my breasts] removed, they really aren't important to me" said they were met with the HCP response, "why would a female not want to have breasts? Let's collectively gawk at the patient until they agree to save them" (non-binary, bisexual, age 37, breast). This resulted in the participant feeling like "it's never going to be safe" and "why couldn't they just listen to me?" HCP lack of understanding of the meaning of gender affirmation, and the interaction of hormonal treatment and cancer treatment was also experienced, with implications for treatment delivery and efficacy (Squires et al., 2022). For example, a trans man told us:

> It is written on my file but staff do not understand what it means, i.e., have I already transitioned or do I want to? … It is a continual issue when blood tests are read and interpreted against male or female ranges. After chemo

and steroids the bone density clinic had trouble working out what a normal reading would be.

(Trans man, queer, 35, uterine)

This lack of awareness of gender-affirming care amongst cancer care professionals makes it difficult for trans patients to make informed medical decisions at the intersection of cancer and gender-affirming healthcare, such as negotiating hormone use during treatment (Taylor & Bryson, 2016; Watters et al., 2015). Conversely, a number of trans cancer survivors talked about everything in their health being attributed to being trans, regardless of the reason for their visit to a HCP, a phenomenon previously described as "trans broken arm syndrome" (Knutson, Koch, Arthur, Mitchell, & Martyr, 2016): "When you say you're trans everything is about being trans, it doesn't matter if you sprained your bloody ankle, everything is because you're trans" (trans man, gay, 55, multiple cancers); "I'm really tired of everyone assuming things are caused by hormones, and that being the #1 thing everyone jumps to when they think of trans cancer patients" (non-binary, queer, 26, ovarian).

Others experience unnecessary or invasive questions from HCPs that are unrelated to the reason for their visit. For example, a trans man reported frequently "being asked lots of intrusive questions about being trans" (trans man, queer, age 34, uterine). Other Out with Cancer Study participants felt that they were "not 'trans' enough" as a non-binary person, "and if I was to share the information a doctor would not understand if I was not seeking to transition into a woman" (non-binary, gay, 35, leukaemia), or told us "The medical profession is always looking for a binary. They're always looking for 'Are you a trans man, trans woman?'. They don't understand the myriad of spaces in between" (non-binary, gay, 32, leukaemia). These accounts suggest that a gender binary is being applied by some HCPs, even when they may be attempting to be trans inclusive (Winter et al., 2016). Others talked of being pathologised when negotiating desired cancer treatment. The decision of a trans participant to have a mastectomy without reconstruction was positioned as a "dysphoric response" by their breast cancer surgeon, who initially refused to do the surgery as a result. Conversely, alternative surgeons the participant was referred to reportedly wanted a "DSM diagnosis [of gender dysphoria]" before they would agree to operate (non-binary, queer, 37, medical intervention and breast), as reported in a previous study (Brown & McElroy, 2018). Either way, trans embodiment and subjectivity is being critically evaluated through a psychiatric lens, based on binary and heteronormative assumptions (Winter et al., 2016).

This misunderstanding, combined with past experiences of hostility and prejudice on the part of HCPs, can lead to non-disclosure of trans identity as a protective mechanism (Ussher, Power, et al., 2022). Only 28.6% of trans Out with Cancer Study participants disclosed their trans identity to all cancer HCPs, with 47.6% selectively disclosing to some HCPs, and 23.8% disclosing to none. As a non-binary queer breast cancer survivor, age 39, told us "I was very scared about my treatment if I told anyone. I already look alternative and even had a normal hair cut when I knew I had surgeries coming up". A non-binary, bisexual breast cancer survivor, age 24, with an intersex variation told us:

> There is so much internalized shame tied into the experience of being in-tersex. It's hard to disclose. I've also disclosed in the past and had medical professionals respond negatively or even Google my variation in front of me. I'm very careful about who I disclose to now.

Non-disclosure served to both "avoid confrontation" and "leverage the system" for trans participants. Fears of confrontation are based in reality, with hostile interac-tions with HCPs reported by a number of trans Out with Cancer Study participants, reflecting previous reports of discrimination towards trans people in healthcare (Shires & Jaffee, 2015). For example, participants told us: "while in hospital I heard them talking about me as if I was a freak being described as high risk need for extra care" (non-binary, gender fluid, 67, pancreatic and prostate):

> I had one therapist in the past … that told me I was unhappy because I wasn't living according to god's will. It's why I hid who I am [in cancer care] because I was so worried about my treatment by others.
>
> *(Non-binary, queer, 39, ovarian)*

This compounds discrimination in broader society: 83.3% of trans participants reported having experienced discrimination for being trans in their life in general. Experiences of HCP discrimination can have a direct impact on trans identity, as a participant told us:

> The discrimination I have experienced from health professionals during my cancer care has reduced my ability to be proud of who I am. This discrimina-tion prevents me from help seeking for my current maintenance care.
>
> *(Non-binary, gender fluid, lesbian/queer, 38, multiple)*

Non-disclosure of trans identity, which for some intersects with LGBQ iden-tity, is an understandable self-protective mechanism. It is notable that accounts of non-disclosure are predominately from non-binary participants, as was the case with cancer carers. Trans people who challenge "the normative coercion to per-form gender dichotomously" (Peters, 2018) have been described as "border-dwell-ers" (Pallotta-Chiarolli, 2010), operating a space in the middle of the gender binary. Non-binary individuals may have greater ability to "pass" as cisgender than other trans people. For example, the experience of a non-binary participant who said "I ride off the privilege of my gender fluidity constantly in order to grin and bear it, and deal with the cis-normativity that it takes to avoid that aspect of discrimination" (queer, 37, breast) contrasts with that of a trans man with ovarian cancer, who told us "You can't hide behind just not telling them [you're trans]" (age 48, straight). However, the ability to pass puts non-binary people at greater risk of diminished sense of self and gender dysphoria (Cole et al., 2002), and can be associated with a burden of secrecy, feelings of anxiety, invisibility, and frustration through the cancer journey (Lisy, Peters, Schofield, & Jefford, 2018). Non-disclosure may thus add to the stress of cancer and result in poor psychological wellbeing (Durso & Meyer, 2013).

Conversely, some trans cancer survivors made a point of disclosing their trans identity to HCPs, wanting to "trail blaze", even though they were "afraid of medical staff treating me more poorly", because they were "not the first, nor will I be the last nonbinary person with a gynaecological cancer" (non-binary, queer, age 35, uterine). Disclosure of sexual orientation and gender identity (SOGI) status to HCPs has positive benefits, including: greater engagement and satisfaction with care, better illness adjustment, and better mental health (Balik et al., 2020; Ruben & Fullerton, 2018).

However, the experience of "coming out repeatedly because of multiple doctors, specialists" when a person is "in pain; very sick; recovering; scared" was described as "absolutely exhausting … no matter how strong I am, how resilient, how proud" (non-binary, bisexual, age 37, breast). The trailblazing participant quoted above also said they were "fucking exhausted" by constant disclosure. However, in contexts where HCPs were trans inclusive – for instance asked for pronouns, included carers in healthcare, and displayed rainbow flags, disclosure was a safer experience, and trans cancer survivors and their partners had a positive experience of cancer care (Ussher, Power, et al., 2022): "I was incredibly worried about how we'd be treated as a queer couple. Turned out that we had no problems at all, but it was horrible that my brain thought of that first" (non-binary, queer, age 34, carer of partner with breast); "Being able to come out and be labelled and addressed [with labels and honorifics] on chemo days or radiation days, makes SUCH a difference" (trans man, queer, 53, thyroid). This demonstrates the vital importance of trans inclusive practices in cancer care, in facilitating the wellbeing of trans patients and their carers (Ussher, Power, et al., 2022).

"Actively excluded from all of the materials": trans exclusion in cancer information and support resources

These negative experiences of participants in the Out with Cancer Study in relation to navigating cancer care are not unique. Previous work with trans people with cancer has highlighted "extraordinary gaps in … the availability of cancer health knowledge", with few patients able to find helpful information about their cancer care, and a particular dearth of trans-specific cancer resources (Taylor & Bryson, 2016). This is in part due to the lack of research on cancer prevalence and experiences in trans populations, which has contributed to uncertainties around contributing risks and appropriate treatment options (Braun et al., 2017; Puechl et al., 2019; Scime, 2019), combined with an absence of initiatives translating what is known into accessible resources. The Out with Cancer Study audited the websites of 69 Australian cancer patient and carer organisations, and found that only 20% included mention of trans people, and only 24% avoided gendered assumptions about cancer types (i.e. only men have prostate cancer, only women have ovarian cancer cancer). This was reflected in comments from our participants:

> It was difficult for me to get appropriate advice relevant to my genital differences. I didn't suffer any further damage as a result, but it added to the stress of the procedure. I also found that advice given assumed I would be heterosexual and having PIV [penis in vagina] sex.
>
> *(Non-binary, queer, age 48, intersex, medical intervention to prevent cancer)*

The intersection of cultural background, gender, and sexuality was also evident in cancer information resources, as a participant said to us, "It's all really white, and white Australian. My partners have not always been white, and they felt actively excluded from all of the materials I brought home for their sexuality, gender and race" (non-binary gender fluid, lesbian/queer, 38 breast, colorectal, ovarian pancreatic).

Trans people may also experience exclusion when seeking experiential information and peer connection with other LGBQTI people with cancer. As is the case with cancer services, trans people are often invisible and erased in peer cancer networks which replicate cis-heterocentric societal dynamics (Squires et al., 2022; Taylor & Bryson, 2016). At the same time, trans support networks tend to focus on gender affirmation processes.[1] As a result, trans people with cancer may have fewer opportunities to connect with and learn from each other in non-specific cancer peer organisations, potentially limiting their access to social support. As one of our survey participants commented:

> All the support networks are directed towards straight older communities. Booklets for careers make awful heteronormative assumptions about gender roles in relationships and provided only anger and frustration rather than comfort to me. The thought of even approaching one of the support groups that catered to this group of people made me feel sick, so I never found any help/peer support.
>
> *(Non-binary, gay, age 34, leukaemia)*

> I have been searching for months for an online community of transgender cancer survivors. To date I haven't found any. As a result, I am going to focus my upcoming Master's of Social Work degree on supports for transgender cancer patients.
>
> *(Trans man, straight, age 48, ovarian)*

Access to cancer services that are informed and sensitive about the needs of trans people are critical; however, they may be hard to locate, or not available (Banerjee, Walters, Staley, Alexander, & Parker, 2018). Many health professionals receive no training on the care of trans patients, and clinicians' lack of knowledge and experience compromises the quality and sensitivity of care received by these populations (Puechl et al., 2019; Ussher, Perz et al., 2022). Turning to the accounts of HCPs can help us to understand why this is so.

"Brush stroke imagining": healthcare professional perspectives on trans inclusive cancer care

Surveys of cancer health professionals have evidenced self-deficits in objective and self-perceived knowledge of the cancer-related needs of trans patients (Banerjee et al., 2018; Schabath et al., 2019; Ussher, Perz et al., 2022). In the Out with Cancer Study, most HCPs reported being comfortable working with LGBTQI patients and were willing to be listed as LGBTQI-friendly professionals, confirming absence of overt prejudice. However, we found significant gaps in HCP knowledge and confidence in the healthcare needs of trans patients, consistent with prior research (Banerjee, Staley, Alexander, Walters, & Parker, 2020; Schabath et al., 2019; Sutter et al., 2020) and lowest confidence with intersex patients, a unique finding of our study. This suggests that the 33% of the Out with Cancer participants who reported intersecting trans and intersex identities are likely to experience multiple marginalisation. Only a small minority of HCPs had received formal education/training on the healthcare needs of trans patients, meaning that "brush stroke imagining" was all HCPs had to rely on. The majority agreed that such education/training should be mandatory for HCPs, in line with previous research (Schabath et al., 2019; Shetty et al., 2016; Sutter et al., 2020).

HCPs' poor knowledge and lack of confidence in working with trans patients contributed to being unsure "if I'm doing the right thing". Demonstrating reflexive awareness of their limited capacities to provide trans inclusive care, HCPs were conscious of having "put my foot in it multiple times", with the potential to "cause offence", "damage rapport", or appear "insensitive". Many HCPs "worried" about asking "stupid" questions and "using the wrong pronoun" because of not having "a great grasp on all of the language and who falls under which bracket" (Ussher, Perz et al., 2022).

> I have no concept about what gender reassignment surgery involves. So I would be lacking in confidence if I was treating somebody who'd been through that. … I would feel very much out of my comfort zone. It would be a steep learning curve for me.
>
> *(Brett, medical practitioner, 37, cis male, gay)*

Consequently, trans people with cancer may receive care that is inadequately informed by or tailored to their needs. Additionally, trans patients report having to teach health professionals about trans healthcare (Kerr et al., 2020). As Out with Cancer Study participants told us, "I always withhold my sexuality [and non-binary identity] if it is someone I won't see again, it's not worth the emotional effort it takes me to educate them" (age 38, lesbian/queer, non-binary gender fluid, breast, colorectal, ovarian pancreatic); "I think people just don't know how to deal with me. What questions to ask; how to ask them" (age 34, queer, non-binary, bladder). Together with health professionals' unintentional and intentional misgendering and referral to trans people using inappropriate language (Ussher, Power et al., 2022), as well as invisibility or ignorance to trans people's chosen support people in cancer care, this may contribute to feelings of distrust and discomfort amongst trans people with cancer and undermine patient–clinician relations (Alpert et al., 2021; Kerr et al., 2020). However, some trans cancer survivors are happy to educate HCPs, and have a positive experience of cancer care as a result:

> I have often been my healthcare professional's FIRST transgender patient/ client. That being said, most of my interactions with those healthcare professionals have been very courteous. They have/had a genuine interest in learning more about transgender care in order to help me further. And I've been happy to help them understand more about it.
>
> *(Trans, straight, 49, ovarian)*

Conclusion

In combination, these patient and carer accounts of increased gender dysphoria and interrupted gender affirmation provide explanation for the association between distress and impact of cancer on trans identity (Ussher, Allison, et al., 2022), suggesting that the very essence of trans embodiment may be disrupted by cancer or cancer caring. However, cancer and cancer treatment can have a positive impact on the embodied identity and lives of some trans people, despite the anxiety and strain of negotiating medical procedures. However, if HCPs operate within a cis-heteronormative framework, and do not understand the meaning of embodied change following cancer treatment for trans individuals, these positive benefits may not be realised. Feelings of gender euphoria will stay within the realm of the individual, and not public, institutional spaces like hospitals, meaning that trans people will need to keep self-policing, or 'splitting' their presentation of self in these spaces.

There is a need for HCPs to be aware of the higher risk of distress of trans cancer survivors and their carers, in particular the intersection of cancer with trans identity and embodiment, difficulties in disclosure of identity and the impact of invisibility in healthcare. HCPs have responsibility for facilitating disclosure with their patients, as many trans patients are too fearful to disclose, or are concerned that they will receive negative responses (Ussher Perz et al., 2022). Specific training in offering trans inclusive and affirmative cancer care as part of basic communication training and ongoing professional development is essential (Pratt-Chapman, 2021; Quinn, Alpert, Sutter, & Schabath, 2020). Such programs can increase HCP confidence, challenge transphobic stereotypes and increase the likelihood of trans patients receiving inclusive and affirmative cancer care. The materiality of the clinical context needs to be improved in order to facilitate disclosure and address trans patient and carer needs. This includes visible indicators of trans inclusivity in clinics, health service websites, and patient support information; acknowledgement of sexual orientation and trans gender identity status on intake forms; and provision of trans-specific information on issues such as sexual health, bodily changes, and the concerns of transgender and intersex people (Alpert et al., 2021; Lisy et al., 2020; Robinson et al., 2020). Providing equitable care to trans cancer patients and their carers is a human rights issue. We know what patients want, and we know the barriers to provision of inclusive and affirmative person- centred trans cancer care. It is time to translate this knowledge into education and training for all oncology HCPs and to ensure there are appropriate and targeted resources and information for trans patients and their carers.

Acknowledgements

The Out with Cancer study was funded by the Australian Research Council Linkage Program grant (LP170100644), the Cancer Council New South Wales, and Prostate Cancer Foundation Australia, with in-kind support provided by National LGBTI Health Alliance, ACON, Breast Cancer Network Australia, Sydney Children's Hospital Network and Canteen. This research was supported by ANZUP and by Register4 through its members' participation in research. We would like to thank our stakeholder advisory group, and all of our LGBTQI carers and HCP participants who volunteered for this study.

Note

1 e.g., https://gendercentre.org.au/support-groups.

References

Alpert, A. B., Gampa, V., Lytle, M. C., Manzano, C., Ruddick, R., Poteat, T., … Kamen, C. S. (2021). I'm not putting on that floral gown: Enforcement and resistance of gender expectations for transgender people with cancer. *Patient Education and Counseling*, *104*(10), 2552–2558.

Austin, A., Papciak, R., & Lovins, L. (2022). Gender euphoria: A grounded theory exploration of experiencing gender affirmation. *Psychology & Sexuality*, 1–21.

Balik, C. H. A., Bilgin, H., Uluman, O. T., Sukut, O., Yilmaz, S., & Buzlu, S. (2020). A systematic review of the discrimination against sexual and gender minority in health care settings. *International Journal of Health Services*, *50*(1), 44–61.

Banerjee, S. C., Staley, J. M., Alexander, K., Walters, C. B., & Parker, P. A. (2020). Encouraging patients to disclose their lesbian, gay, bisexual, or transgender (LGBT) status: oncology health care providers' perspectives. *Translational Behavioral Medicine*, *10*, 918–927.

Banerjee, S. C., Walters, C. B., Staley, J. M., Alexander, K., & Parker, P. A. (2018). knowledge, beliefs, and communication behavior of oncology health-care providers (HCPs) regarding lesbian, gay, bisexual, and transgender (LGBT) patient health care. *Journal of Health Communication*, *23*(4), 329–339.

Boehmer, U., Gereige, J., Winter, M., Ozonoff, A., & Scout, N. (2020). Transgender individuals' cancer survivorship: Results of a cross-sectional study. *Cancer*, *126*(12), 2829–2836.

Braun, H., Nash, R., Tangpricha, V., Brockman, J., Ward, K., & Goodman, M. (2017). Cancer in transgender people: Evidence and methodological considerations. *Epidemiologic Reviews, 39*(1), 93–107.

Brown, G. R., & Jones, K. T. (2015). Incidence of breast cancer in a cohort of 5,135 transgender veterans. *Breast Cancer Research and Treatment, 149*(1), 191–198.

Brown, M. T., & McElroy, J. A. (2018). Sexual and gender minority breast cancer patients choosing bilateral mastectomy without reconstruction: "I now have a body that fits me". *Women & Health, 58*(4), 403–418.

Clements-Nolle, K., Marx, R., & Katz, M. (2006). Attempted suicide among transgender persons: The influence of gender-based discrimination and victimization. *Journal of homosexuality, 51*(3), 53–70.

Cole, S., Denny, D., Eyler, A., & Samons, S. (2002). Issues of transgender. In S. Levine (Ed.), *Psychological perspectives on human sexuality* (pp. 149–195). Washington, DC: American Psychiatric Association.

Connolly, D., Hughes, X., & Berner, A. (2020). Barriers and facilitators to cervical cancer screening among transgender men and non-binary people with a cervix: A systematic narrative review. *Preventive Medicine, 135*, 106071–106071.

Crenshaw, K. (1991). Mapping the margins: Intersectionality, identity politics, and violence against women of color. *Stanford Law Review, 43*(6), 1241–1299.

Deebel, N. A., Morin, J. P., Autorino, R., Vince, R., Grob, B., & Hampton, L. J. (2017). Prostate cancer in transgender women: Incidence, etiopathogenesis, and management challenges. *Urology, 110*, 166–171.

Durso, L., & Meyer, I. (2013). Patterns and predictors of disclosure of sexual orientation to healthcare providers among lesbians, gay men, and bisexuals. *Sexuality Research and Social Policy, 10*(1), 35–42.

Foster, C. R. (2021). Here's what makes top surgery different from a mastectomy. Retrieved from www.allure.com/story/top-surgery-mastectomy-difference

Graham, I. D., Logan, J., Harrison, M. B., Straus, S. E., Tetroe, J., Caswell, W., & Robinson, N. (2006). Lost in knowledge translation: Time for a map? *Journal of Continuing Education in the Health Professions, 26*(1), 13–24.

Grant, J., Mottet, L., & Tanis, J. (2011). *Injustice at every turn: A report of the National Transgender Discrimination Survey.* Washington, DC.

Hawkey, A. J., & Ussher, J. M. (2022). Feminist research: Inequality, social change, and intersectionality. In U. Flick (Ed.), *The Sage handbook of qualitative research design* (vol. 1, pp. 175–193). London: Sage.

Ingham, M. D., Lee, R. J., MacDermed, D., & Olumi, A. F. (2018). Prostate cancer in transgender women. *Urologic Oncology, 36*(12), 518–525.

Jackson, S. S., Nambiar, K. Z., O'Callaghan, S., & Berner, A. M. (2022). Understanding the role of sex hormones in cancer for the transgender community. *Trends in Cancer, 8*(4), 273–275.

James, S. E., Herman, J. L., Rankin, S., Keisling, M., Mottet, L., & Anafi, M. (2016). *The Report of the 2015 U.S. Transgender Survey.* In N. C. F. T. Equality (Ed.). Washington, DC.

Jiang, D. D., Gallagher, S., Burchill, L., Berli, J., & Dugi, D., 3rd. (2019). Implementation of a Pelvic Floor Physical Therapy Program for Transgender Women Undergoing Gender-Affirming Vaginoplasty. *Obstetrics & Gynecology, 133*(5), 1003–1011.

Johnson, M. J., Nemeth, L. S., Mueller, M., Eliason, M. J., & Stuart, G. W. (2016). Qualitative study of cervical cancer screening among lesbian and bisexual women and transgender men. *Cancer Nursing, 39*(6), 455–463.

Kerr, L., Fisher, C., & Jones, T. (2019). TRANScending discrimination in health & cancer care: A study of trans & gender diverse Australians *ARCSHS Monograph Series No. 117*: La Trobe University.

Kerr, L., Fisher, C. M., & Jones, T. (2020). "I'm not from another planet": The alienating cancer care experiences of trans and gender-diverse people. *Cancer Nursing, 44*(6), E438–E446.

Knutson, D., Koch, J. M., Arthur, T., Mitchell, T. A., & Martyr, M. A. (2016). "Trans broken arm": Health care stories from transgender people in rural areas. *Journal of Research on Women and Gender, 7*(1), 30–46.

Levitt, H. M., & Ippolito, M. R. (2014). Being transgender: Navigating minority stressors and developing authentic self-presentation. *Psychology of Women Quarterly, 38*(1), 46–64.

Lisy, K., Hulbert-Williams, N., Ussher, J. M., Alpert, A., Kamen, C., & Jefford, M. (2020). Lesbian, gay, bisexual and transgender issues. In M. Watson & D. Kissane (Eds.), *Sexual health, fertility and relationships in cancer care.* Oxford: Oxford University Press.

Lisy, K., Peters, M. D. J., Schofield, P., & Jefford, M. (2018). Experiences and unmet needs of lesbian, gay, and bisexual people with cancer care: A systematic review and meta-synthesis. *Psycho-oncology (Chichester, UK), 27*(6), 1480–1489.

Marecek, J. (2016). Invited reflection: Intersectionality theory and feminist psychology. *Psychology of Women Quarterly, 40*(2), 177–181.

Nuttbrock, L. A., Bockting, W. O., Hwahng, S., Rosenblum, A., Mason, M., Macri, M., & Becker, J. (2009). Gender identity affirmation among male-to-female transgender persons: A life course analysis across types of relationships and cultural/lifestyle factors. *Sexual and Relationship Therapy: Gender Variance and Transgender Identity, 24*(2), 108–125.

Oladeru, O. T., Ma, S. J., Miccio, J. A., Wang, K., Attwood, K., Singh, A. K., … Neira, P. M. (2022). Breast and cervical cancer screening disparities in transgender people. *American Journal of Clinical Oncology, 45*(3), 116–121.

Pallotta-Chiarolli, M. (2010). *Border sexualities: Border families in schools.* New York: Rowman & Littlefield.

Peitzmeier, S. M., Reisner, S. L., Harigopal, P., & Potter, J. (2014). Female-to-male patients have high prevalence of unsatisfactory paps compared to non-transgender females: Implications for cervical cancer screening. *Journal of General Internal Medicine: JGIM, 29*(5), 778–784.

Perz, J., Ussher, J. M., Butow, P., & Wain, G. (2011). Gender differences in cancer carer psychological distress: an analysis of moderators and mediators. *European Journal of Cancer Care, 20*(5), 610–619.

Peters, J. (2018). *A feminist post-transsexual autoethnography: Challenging normative gender coercion.* London: Routledge.

Power, R., Ussher, J. M., Perz, J., Allison, K., Hawkey, A. J., & Team, T. O. W. C. S. (2022). "Surviving discrimination by pulling together": LGBTQI cancer patient and carer experiences of minority stress and social support. *Frontiers in Oncology, 12,* 918016. https://doi.org/10.3389/fonc.2022.918016

Pratt-Chapman, M. L. (2021). Efficacy of LGBTQI cultural competency training for oncology social workers. *Journal of Psychosocial Oncology, 39*(1), 135–142.

Pratt-Chapman, M. L., Alpert, A. B., & Castillo, D. A. (2021). Health outcomes of sexual and gender minorities after cancer: A systematic review. *Systematic Reviews, 10,* 183.

Puechl, A. M., Russell, K., & Gray, B. A. (2019). Care and cancer screening of the transgender population. *Journal of Women's Health (Larchmont), 28*(6), 761–768.

Quinn, G. P., Alpert, A. B., Sutter, M., & Schabath, M. B. (2020). What oncologists should know about treating sexual and gender minority patients with cancer. *JCO Oncology Practice, 16*(6), 309–316.

Robinson, K. H., Townley, C., Ullman, J., Denson, N., Davies, C., Bansel, P., … Lambert, S. (2020). *Advancing LGBTQ+ safety and inclusion: Understanding the lived experiences and health needs of sexuality and gender diverse people in Greater Western Sydney.* Sydney: Western Sydney University and ACON.

Ruben, M. A., & Fullerton, M. (2018). Proportion of patients who disclose their sexual orientation to healthcare providers and its relationship to patient outcomes: A meta-analysis and review. *Patient Education and Counseling, 101*(9), 1549–1560.

Rubin, L. R., & Tanenbaum, M. (2011). "Does that make me a woman?" Breast cancer, mastectomy, and breast reconstruction decisions among sexual minority women. *Psychology of Women Quarterly, 35*(3), 401–414.

Schabath, M. B., Blackburn, C. A., Sutter, M. E., Kanetsky, P. A., Vadaparampil, S. T., Simmons, V. N., ... Quinn, G. P. (2019). National survey of oncologists at National Cancer Institute-designated comprehensive cancer centers: Attitudes, knowledge, and practice behaviors about LGBTQ patients with cancer. *Journal of Clinical Oncology, 37*(7), 547–558.

Scime, S. (2019). Inequities in cancer care among transgender people: Recommendations for change. *Canadian Oncology Nursing Journal = Revue Canadienne de Nursing Oncologique, 29*(2), 87–91.

Shetty, G., Sanchez, J. A., Lancaster, J. M., Wilson, L. E., Quinn, G. P., & Schabath, M. B. (2016). Oncology healthcare providers' knowledge, attitudes, and practice behaviors regarding LGBT health. *Patient Education and Counseling, 99*(10), 1676–1684.

Shires, D. A., & Jaffee, K. (2015). Factors associated with health care discrimination experiences among a national sample of female-to-male transgender individuals. *Health & Social Work, 40*(2), 134–141.

Sinding, C., Grassau, P., & Barnoff, L. (2007). Community support, community values: The experiences of lesbians diagnosed with cancer. *Women & Health, 44*(2), 59–79.

Squires, L. R., Bilash, T., Kamen, C. S., & Garland, S. N. (2022). Psychosocial needs and experiences of transgender and gender diverse people with cancer: A scoping review and recommendations for improved research and care. *LGBT Health, 9*(1), 8–17.

Sutter, M. E., Bowman-Curci, M. L., Duarte Arevalo, L. F., Sutton, S. K., Quinn, G. P., & Schabath, M. B. (2020). A survey of oncology advanced practice providers' knowledge and attitudes towards sexual and gender minorities with cancer. *Journal of Clinical Nursing, 29*(15–16), 2953–2966.

Taylor, E. T., & Bryson, M. K. (2016). Cancer's margins: Trans★ and gender nonconforming people's access to knowledge, experiences of cancer health, and decision-making. *LGBT Health, 3*(1), 79–89.

Tolman, D. L., Bowman, C. P., & Fahs, B. (2014). Sexuality and embodiment. In D. L. Tolman & L. M. Diamond (Eds.), *APA handbook of sexuality and psychology: Vol. 1. Person-based approaches* (pp. 759–804). Washington, DC: American Psychological Association.

Ussher, J. M., Allison, K., Perz, J., Power, R., & The Out with Cancer Study Team. (2022). LGBTQI cancer patients' quality of life and distress: A comparison by gender, sexuality, age, cancer type and geographical remoteness. *Frontiers in Oncology*, doi.org/10.3389/fonc.2022.873642

Ussher, J. M., Perz, J., Allison, K., Power, R., Hawkey, A., Dowsett, G. W., ... Anazodo, A. (2022). Attitudes, knowledge and practice behaviours of oncology health care professionals towards lesbian, gay, bisexual, transgender, queer and intersex (LGBTQI) patients and their carers: A mixed-methods study. *Patient Education and Counseling, 105*(7), 2512–2523.

Ussher, J. M., Perz, J., Rose, D., Dowsett, G. W., Chambers, S., Williams, S., ... Latini, D. (2017). Threat of sexual disqualification: The consequences of erectile dysfunction and other sexual changes for gay and bisexual men with prostate cancer. *Archives of Sexual Behavior, 46*(7), 2043–2057.

Ussher, J. M., Power, R., Perz, J., Hawkey, A. J., Allison, K., & The Out with Cancer Study Team. (2022). LGBTQI inclusive cancer care: A discourse analytic study of health care professional, patient and carer perspectives. *Frontiers in Oncology, 12*, 832657. doi: 10.3389/fonc.2022.832657.

Wandrey, R. L., Qualls, W. D., & Mosack, K. E. (2016). Rejection of breast reconstruction among lesbian breast cancer patients. *LGBT Health*, *3*(1), 74–78.

Warner, L. R. (2008). A best practices guide to intersectional approaches in psychological research. *Sex Roles*, *59*(5–6), 454–463.

Watters, Y., Harsh, J., & Corbett, C. (2015). Cancer care for transgender patients: Systematic literature review. *International Journal of Transgenderism*, *15*(3–4), 136–145.

Winter, S., Diamond, M., Green, J., Karasic, D., Reed, T., Whittle, S., & Wylie, K. (2016). Transgender people: Health at the margins of society. *The Lancet*, *388*(10042), 390–400.

8

VIEWS ON FERTILITY PRESERVATION AMONGST TRANS YOUNG PEOPLE AND THEIR PARENTS

Damien W. Riggs and Clare Bartholomaeus

Introduction

Since the release of the World Professional Association for Transgender Health's *Standards of Care 7* in 2011, there has been a marked growth in attention to, and recognition of, the reproductive rights of trans people. In the *Standards of Care 7*, only two pages were devoted to reproductive health, reflecting the relative dearth of attention to reproductive justice for trans people up to that point, and indeed reflecting what was at the time a much wider number of countries that mandated sterilisation as part of legal gender transition. Since then, shifts in awareness of the rights of trans people to reproduce have translated into a growing body of research evidence focused on trans people's experiences of reproduction, including specifically with regard to fertility preservation (e.g., Adeleye et al., 2019; Armaund et al., 2017; Bartholomaeus & Riggs, 2020; Riggs & Bartholomaeus, 2018a). This includes coverage of fertility and fertility preservation in health and medical guidelines for trans children and young people (e.g., Oliphant et al., 2018; Telfer et al., 2017), and an advocacy movement focused on ensuring reproductive justice for trans people (e.g., Pro-Choice Public Education Project and LGBT Community Centre, n.d.).

Depending on the country and jurisdiction, fertility preservation may be offered as a matter of course for trans people as a part of medical gender transition, or it may be seen as a specialist or exceptional case. Fertility preservation may be covered by social healthcare in some contexts, or it may be user-pays. The most common form of fertility preservation available for trans people is the storage of gametes, which can occur either ideally before the commencement of gender affirming hormone therapies, or if such therapies are ceased at any point. Some gender-affirming surgeries, such as orchiectomy or oophorectomy, will mean that fertility preservation is no longer possible. For people who decide to undertake fertility preservation, in

DOI: 10.4324/9781003138310-8

many contexts there will be ongoing costs associated with the storage of gametes, and in some contexts there may be limits to how long stored gametes are considered viable (Riggs & Bartholomaeus, 2018a).

Reflecting the life course approach introduced in the first chapter of this book, research and advocacy in relation to fertility preservation for trans people has increasingly focused on children and young people. Such a focus was noticeably absent from the *Standards of Care 7*, likely reflecting the fact that at the time they were published far fewer children were able to access gender affirming medical care, and thus far fewer were likely to find their fertility impacted by treatment. In the ten-year period since the release of the *Standards of Care 7*, referrals to paediatric gender clinics have grown exponentially. For example, in Australia, paediatric services have reported an increase from a very small number of young people seeking services at the start of the millennium, to over 200 referrals per year presently at individual clinics (Telfer, Tollit, & Feldman, 2015). In the United States, paediatric services have reported a similar increase from small numbers in 2015 to over 200 in 2017 at individual clinics (Handler et al., 2019). Paediatric services in each of the four Nordic countries have reported increases from very small numbers in 2010 to between 150 and 350 referrals in 2017, and services across the United Kingdom have reported increases from very small numbers in 2010 to upwards of 2000 referrals in 2017 (Kaltiala et al., 2020). Finally, paediatric services across Canada have reported an increase from very small numbers in 2010 to over 1000 in 2016 (Bauer et al., 2018). It is important to note that the increase in young people presenting at services is likely to reflect higher rates of disclosure and seeking of medical services, rather than implying that trans young people did not exist previously.

Given that in many contexts trans young people now commence medical treatment (such as puberty suppressants) at younger ages, the topic of fertility preservation is especially fraught. For young people who have not commenced the puberty associated with their assigned sex, in some contexts storage of tissue from the reproductive glands is offered, although this treatment is experimental and does not yet offer the possibility for creating life from the stored tissue. For young people who have already commenced puberty the storage of gametes may be possible, but is likely to be distressing for many young people. The topic of fertility preservation for trans young people thus raises complicated questions about reproductive justice. Pronatalist assumptions may mean that all children – and especially children assigned female at birth, given mandates to motherhood for people assigned female – are expected to one day want to be parents (of genetically related children), and thus should all be required to undertake fertility preservation. There is also increasing family diversity where parenting is undertaken (and largely accepted) in many forms. At the same time, and given cisgenderist assumptions, trans young people may be seen as less-than-fit future parents, and thus may not be offered fertility preservation. It is also important to recognise that any desire to preserve fertility may sit in tension with the desire to receive timely access to affirming medical care. And, finally, even if young people do undertake fertility preservation, there is no guarantee that stored tissue or gametes will translate into conception in the future, and the costs associated with fertility preservation can be a significant barrier for some young people and their parents.

In this chapter we take up the topic of fertility preservation for trans young people. We report on survey data collected with Australian parents of trans young people, and dyadic interviews undertaken with trans young people and their parents. In focusing on the views of young people and their parents, our interest is to explore some of the tensions outlined above, with a specific focus on some of the conceptual frameworks introduced in the first chapter of this book, specifically with regard to pronatalism, temporality, and cisgenderism. In so doing, we consider how affirming approaches to clinical care for trans young people sit alongside a complexity of issues associated with reproductive justice for trans young people. We thus conclude the chapter by considering how a reproductive justice approach may inform fertility preservation for trans young people into the future.

Literature overview and project background

Much of the initial research on trans young people and fertility preservation involved retrospective case reports, examining rates of fertility preservation, particularly in the United States (e.g., Chen et al., 2017; Nahata et al., 2017). This literature suggested relatively low rates of fertility preservation. Importantly, while most of the young people included in these studies had been offered fertility preservation and provided with counselling on the topic, few availed themselves of the possibility. Reasons given included prohibitive cost, dysphoria associated with the idea of storing gametes, no desire to have a (genetically related) child in the future, and a desire to proceed immediately with gender-affirming medical treatment. This initial literature did not focus on the question of reproductive justice, though did raise concerns about the decision-making capacity of trans young people, highlighting the spectre of developmentalism and pronatalism that often frames discussions about trans young people and fertility (Riggs & Bartholomaeus, 2020).

Subsequent interview and survey research, again primarily conducted in the United States, has expanded understandings of fertility preservation for trans young people. Some studies have reported that young people experience the perception of pronatalism on the part of medical professionals, particularly those who strongly encourage or require fertility preservation (Chen et al., 2018). This is especially the case for trans young people who were assigned female at birth, highlighting the intersections of cisgenderism and pronatalism (i.e., that pronatalism is especially directed towards those who are potentially capable of gestation). It is important to note that this injunction to fertility preservation for people assigned female at birth sits in contrast to a perception reported among medical professionals that fertility preservation for this group of people is inherently more challenging or difficult than it is for people assigned male (Riggs & Bartholomaeus, 2020). Yet, despite this perception, some trans people assigned female are strongly encouraged to undertake fertility preservation.

Other studies have similarly highlighted the effects of cisgenderism, specifically with regard to normative assumptions about bodies and reproduction. In some studies, young people have reported the wish that their gametes normatively reflected their gender, and that gametes that were seen to instead reflect assigned sex were viewed as distressing and undesirable in terms of fertility preservation (e.g., Kyweluk, Sajwani, & Chen, 2018). This led some young people in these studies to create imagined futures in which forms of reproduction were possible that reflected their gender rather than their assigned sex, such as uterine transplants for trans girls and young women. Absent of these imaginaries being medical possibilities at present, other studies report that young people chose to eschew fertility preservation, so as not to have stored gametes that they felt were not reflective of their gender (e.g., Harris, Kolaitis, & Frader, 2020; Persky et al., 2020). This includes young people who felt that they would struggle to see themselves as adopting a particular parenting role (i.e., a mother or a father), because they held deterministic views about the cultural meanings attributed to gametes (i.e., that conceiving a child using one's stored sperm would make it culturally difficult to claim the role of mother). These findings again highlight how cisgenderism shapes trans young people's decision making about fertility preservation.

Previous research has also explored the extent to which parents of trans young people may view fertility preservation as desirable. Some young people have reported coercion by their parents, such that they would not support gender affirming medical care if fertility preservation was not undertaken (e.g., Chen et al., 2019). Other studies suggest more implicit forms of pronatalism, such as in the suggestion that a parent accepting that a child did not want to have children in the future required 'letting go of a dream' held by parents (e.g., Harris et al., 2020). As noted above, there is a normative assumption that trans young people are too young to make decisions about fertility preservation. Yet, in the face of strong expectations from others, including both parents and medical professionals, some trans young people are still able to assert their views. Such views likely reflect a complex set of interplays between their experiences of their gender, their views on the meaning of gametes, and their imagined reproductive futures.

With regard to the views of parents specifically, previous research suggests, and again contrary to developmentalist concerns, that many parents believe that a child is capable of making a meaningful decision about future fertility (e.g., Persky et al., 2020). For such parents, research suggests that some parents have a clear understanding of why fertility preservation may not be desirable for their child, especially if children view gametes as reflecting their assigned sex as opposed to their gender (Harris et al., 2020). Nonetheless, parent views may still potentially be at odds with those of their children in some families. Some parents may believe that their children should delay gender affirming treatments in order to undertake fertility preservation (Persky et al., 2020). Some parents may also be less likely to view the gendering of gametes as creating a conflict for trans young people. In other words, some parents may not understand why a child considers the storage of gametes to be dysphoria-inducing, which is reflected in the fact that some parents may often not take dysphoria into account when making decisions about fertility preservation (Persky et al., 2020).

In this chapter we draw on data from two separate projects. The first was a survey of Australian parents of trans young people, focused on the topic of fertility preservation (further details about this project are available in Riggs & Bartholomaeus, 2020). All of the 78 parent participants were women, and most were heterosexual and in a relationship. Children ranged in age from 4 to 29 years ($M = 13.90$, $SD = 5.49$). Of the parent participants' children, 52.6% were girls, 41.0% were boys, and 6.4% were non-binary, as reported by parents. Parent participants responded to items asking about fertility preservation for their child, including in terms of undertaking fertility preservation, decision making about fertility preservation, and experiences of fertility preservation (if applicable). Conventional content analysis was used to analyse open-ended questions (Hsieh & Shannon, 2005).

The second project involved dyadic interviews with Australian trans young people and their parents (further details about this study are available in Bartholomaeus, Riggs & Pullen Sansfaçon, 2020; Riggs, Bartholomaeus & Pullen Sansfaçon, 2021). Ten interviews were conducted, nine with one parent and child, and one with two parents and child. The young people participating ranged in age from 11 to 17 years ($M = 14.3$). Of the young people participating, five reported their gender as male, four as female, and one as male and female or non-binary. Of the parent participants, nine reported their gender as female, one as male, and one as non-binary. The interviews focused on gender-affirming care, with one question focused specifically on fertility preservation and another on fertility more broadly. All responses to fertility and fertility preservation were analysed thematically and key themes were developed (Braun & Clarke, 2006).

Parent survey responses

Of the parent participants, 47% said their child had indicated a desire to be a parent in the future. Children who had expressed to their parents a desire to be a parent in the future were statistically more likely to be older. In terms of how their child might become a parent in the future, a majority of parent participants reported that their child was unsure how they might become a parent, with the next most common response being adoption. In terms of undertaking fertility preservation, 17% of the participants indicated that their child had done so, with the most common form being storing gametes. For participants whose child had undertaken fertility preservation, all but one had received counselling prior to this. In terms of who had undertaken fertility preservation, trans girls and young women were those statistically more likely to have done so.

Further, in terms of participants whose children had undertaken fertility preservation, in response to an open-ended question about who made the decision, the greatest number of participants reported that they had made the decision (e.g., "My child was not really interested, but I talked her into it"). The next most common responses were the child making the decision (e.g., "My child really wants to be able to have children one day, so that was important to her and we wanted her to have that option in her future"), or the decision being required by professionals (e.g., "It was a requirement of accessing puberty blockers by the endocrinologist"). The majority of participants reported that their child had a positive experience of fertility preservation (e.g., "The clinic was very understanding, used her correct name, had honest but sensitive conversations about the process"), though a minority reported negative experiences (e.g., "The process was very distressing for my child as she was misgendered by the fertility storage centre").

As noted above, for the majority of participants their child had not undertaken fertility preservation. For a majority of these participants, their open-ended responses indicated that the decision was still pending, either due to prohibitive costs, not being aware that fertility preservation was an option, needing more information, or the child being too young. For those who had already made an active decision for their child not to undertake fertility preservation, three common reasons were given by participants: (1) that they had received advice from a medical professional that their child could choose to conceive at a later point, (2) that their child was not willing to delay gender affirming treatment in order to undertake fertility preservation, and (3) that their child was clear they did not want to be a parent in the future.

Child and parent interviews

In this section we explore the fertility preservation perspectives of both children and their parents from our dyadic interviews. The key themes relating to fertility preservation identified from the interviews were: (1) normative gendering of bodies, gametes, and parenting roles, (2) accounts of pronatalism; (3) restrictions on the availability of options, (4) temporality and the passage of time, and (5) fertility preservation and an imagined future.

Normative gendering of bodies, gametes, and parenting role

In this first theme we explore participant accounts of bodies, gametes, and parenting roles that evoke normative assumptions that are cisgenderist. For example, language typically associated with assigned sex was often utilised to refer to puberty and gametes, as evident in the following extract:

> JASMINE (AGE 13): For the thing about me needing to go through male puberty, basically, I don't want to do that.
> LIZ (MOTHER OF JASMINE): Yeah, and you'd been required to go a fair way into male puberty in order to collect sperm as well. So those are the two aspects that we're looking at, the two reasons one might want to go through a bit of male puberty first, and it's a definite no from Jasmine on both counts.

Certainly our suggestion here is not that Jasmine should have wanted to go through a puberty associated with her assigned sex. Rather, our suggestion is that conversations about fertility preservation, as was the case for the extract above, may be limiting and potentially distressing when language associated with assigned sex is used (e.g. 'male puberty', 'sperm'). Certainly, some other participants indicated that when such normative language was used by fertility specialists, it led to participants 'switching off' from the information they were receiving, thus potentially compromising their capacity to give informed consent (i.e., when language associated with assigned sex was used, participants reported that they disengaged from the information relayed to them).

In another interview a young person, in conversation with her parent, challenged the use of cisgenderist language in regard to potential future parenting roles:

> DENISE (MOTHER OF AMELIE): If you decide to go in a female direction and you get female hormones and you even get surgery down the track, what about the idea of when you're in your 20s and suddenly go "I'd really love to be a parent. A father" using your sperm, like what – how does this –
>
> AMELIE (AGE 12): Why would I be a father?
>
> DENISE: Because you're physically a male, so you'd be sperm induced.
>
> AMELIE: I'd be a mother.
>
> DENISE: Oh yeah, no. You're right.
>
> AMELIE: I wouldn't be a father, I'd be a mother.
>
> DENISE: I actually stand corrected. Yeah, you're right.

Here Denise equates gametes, and specifically sperm, with fathering, and moreover reiterates the assumption that this equates with being 'physically a male'. Amelie challenges this normative understanding, instead asserting that regardless of how gametes might be normatively understood by others, Amelie would be a mother. Obviously this conversation ended in a positive direction, with Denise conceding that her normative assumptions were incorrect. However, it is possible to imagine how differently the conversation might have gone had Denise continued to insist upon a normatively gendered understanding of gametes, embodiment, and parenting roles. What this exchange also highlights is the impact of normative gendered assumptions, and the need for parents to consciously change their way of thinking and talking in order to support their child.

Accounts of pronatalism

As we have written about elsewhere (e.g., Riggs & Bartholomaeus, 2020), pronatalism is at times evident when some medical professionals assume that all trans people will want to have children, and more specifically, that they will want to have children to whom they are genetically related. For Jasmine, there was certainly the perception that the fertility specialist she saw was intent upon her undertaking fertility preservation, despite this not being of particular interest to her:

> JASMINE (AGE 13): [Fertility specialist] was very adamant about me going through male puberty to the extent that I could get the sperm. I don't know why, he just had a very strong opinion that there's no other way. Again, there probably is no other way …

INTERVIEWER: … to have children that are genetically related to you, or did he just think children at all?

JASMINE: He just meant genetically related, but I don't care if they're genetically related or not.

LIZ (MOTHER OF JASMINE): And nothing was more important to Jasmine at that point than not having her voice break, which was a fundamental part of getting the sperm. He just, he couldn't seem to see through that. I understand. He's a fertility specialist. He looks through a prism of fertility. Fine, but not everyone who sees you is there because that's their number one goal, so he could've worded it differently.

As Jasmine notes, having children who were genetically related to her was not a concern, yet despite this, Jasmine felt that the fertility specialist attempted to pressure her to go through the puberty associated with her assigned sex in order to store gametes. Liz makes an interesting additional point, namely that the fertility specialist could only see 'through the prism of fertility' as that was the area he specialised in. As we have explored elsewhere (Riggs, 2019), the assumption that fertility only pertains to utilising one's gametes to conceive a child creates a very narrow conceptualisation of potential future parenthood, in effect precluding the exploration of other potential pathways to parenthood, such as adoption, fostering, or donor conception. Certainly, many of our participants indicated that should they decide to become a parent in the future, adoption would be the most appealing option, echoing previous research with young people (e.g., Chen et al., 2018; Chiniara et al., 2019; Nahata et al., 2017).

For other families, it would appear that pronatalism informed the views of parents when it came to the topic of fertility preservation, as much as they were supportive of their children:

JULES (MOTHER OF MILES): For [husband] and I, I would be really sad to see Miles do anything that – again, I guess, because Miles's always said that he wouldn't do anything until 18, it hasn't been a huge issue. And I know I would be really sad to see Miles do things that would mean that he couldn't have babies, but if that was the way that it went, that's the way it went. But when people have said to us, "Well, what's he going to do about babies one day?" It's like, he's 13. Nobody is asking whether my 16-year-old is going to have a baby one day.

MILES (AGE 13): Yes. I don't like the idea. I don't like the idea of sex in general. I'm repulsed by it.

JULES: Somebody else could have the baby. It was always your plan that if you did have a baby, I was going to live next door so I could change its nappies.

In this extract Jules is quite clear that she would be 'sad' if her son made decisions prior to turning 18 that prevented him from 'having babies'. Yet this sadness stands in direct contrast to the later statement that Miles is 13, and that 'nobody is asking whether my [cisgender] 16-year-old is going to have a baby one day'. On the one hand, Jules finds it atypical for children to be expected to consider future parenthood desires, yet on the other hand she has already implicitly determined that Miles shouldn't make decisions that would preclude future parenthood. We would suggest that both developmentalism and pronatalism mediate these contradictory positions: that children can't be expected to know what they want in the future, but that ultimately they should be expected to want (genetically related) children. This is despite Miles making a statement that is potentially both trans-specific and may also be true for other (cisgender) children his age, namely the idea of sex being 'repulsive'. This statement may reflect that he was talking in front of his mother, may reflect an age-specific understanding of sex, but certainly may also reflect his views about intercourse as a trans boy.

By contrast to the extract above, in some conversations between children and their parents, normative assumptions were named and explored:

> AMELIE (AGE 12): It's really like are you okay with not maybe having – I'm sorry, but never being a grandparent?
> DENISE (MOTHER OF AMELIE): I'm fine with that, thank you.
> AMELIE: Well, you'll still be a grandparent, but you won't be genetically related
> DENISE: I'm fine with that, thank you.

Here Amelie appears to treat it as axiomatic that her mother would want grandchildren to whom she is genetically related. Given the types of conversations that occurred in other interviews, such as that in the previous extract, it is readily evident that trans young people are aware of pronatalism and are aware that they need to consider how this may impact them and their parents. While Denise expressed that she was not concerned about genetic relatedness, Amelie still reinforces that Denise would be a grandparent (i.e., that Amelie will still potentially have children in some way), thus adhering to a pronatalist narrative, even if challenging some of its normative assumptions with regard to genetic relatedness.

Restrictions on the availability of options

As we discussed in the introduction to this chapter, fertility preservation can be especially fraught for trans young people who have not gone through the puberty associated with their assigned sex. This highlights a tension between reproductive justice and the medical options available that might allow someone to enact reproductive rights. Some young people and their parents, for example, had attempted to explore options for fertility preservation, only to find that they were not available in their home state:

LIZ (MOTHER OF JASMINE): We tried to look into getting a testicular biopsy for Jasmine, which is an experimental thing that's being …

JASMINE (AGE 13): It seemed like a good idea.

LIZ: It's being offered at [interstate hospital]. The week that we got our referral, and someone else in our circle got their referral as well, that hospital sent out an email saying, "We won't take referrals from interstate". Which is an issue, as in [local hospital] document it suggests looking into fertility preservation, and they mention testicular biopsy. I wrote back to them and I said, "That's great, but you're not offering it". So if the hospital here would offer that, even if it's experimental, at least we would have the option to do something.

Here Liz highlights the differences between hospitals being aware that there are a range of options, and those options actually being available to young people. In a sense, this is a very clear issue of reproductive justice: that an experimental treatment is available more broadly, but not in a specific context. To have that possibility raised, only to be quashed, demonstrates a serious limitation to reproductive justice for some trans young people, as the following extract similarly notes:

AMANDA (PARENT OF ASHLEIGH, AGE 15): We had an appointment and everything [to discuss tissue storage locally] and then they cancelled the appointment and it turns out that they haven't got the facilities to store the tissue. So stuff like that has been frustrating, where you think, "well if you lived in a different state you would get this". So we felt sad about that for quite a while and then I actually randomly read an article online saying the person who developed that procedure isn't holding out much hope that anything much will come of it.

For Amanda, not only had they been told about the possibility of tissue storage (as was also the case for Liz and Jasmine), but they had gone as far as to make an appointment. For Amanda this was akin to a sliding doors moment: that, had they lived in a different state, they might well have proceeded with tissue storage. Amanda appears to have found a way to reconcile this outcome by emphasising that tissue storage doesn't 'hold out much hope'. Yet this does not mean that Amanda's daughter was not effectively excluded from making a purposive decision about fertility preservation. Rather, Amanda's daughter was excluded by the option not being medically available.

Temporality and the passage of time

As was explored in the first chapter of this book, temporality for trans people can take quite specific forms, given waiting times for medical treatment, and also as a product of gender transition, through which past and future narratives may shift. For trans young people and their parents, specifically in the context of fertility preservation, the passage of time and the experience of temporality can hold unique meanings:

> KRISTINA (PARENT OF MARIAH, AGE 17): One thing I would definitely say to other parents, is that you might feel that your child is on the cusp of, any day, their voice is going to break. And that may be the case, but it actually is spread out through a few months. You do have the time [as puberty starts]. This is spread out through years, and you do have the time. And even though that urgency is there, and you feel it from your child that they're feeling that anxiousness and you just want to help them, but the best thing is to just sit back and just slow the process and work with your professionals.
>
> [...]
>
> MARC (FATHER OF MARIAH): And it's a massive thing for someone, a teenager, to start thinking about fertility at such a young age.
>
> [...]
>
> KRISTINA: I think it was a real eyeopener to us that this is, for someone so young to make a decision about their fertility and preserving it, which is not for everyone, but there was like a moment where we were all just, Mariah's 100 per cent on this road and in her journey.

For Kristina, temporality with regard to fertility preservation is marked concurrently by both urgency and a more gradual passage of time. Of the two, Kristina emphasises the importance of parents taking their time to make decisions, at the same time as acknowledging that this is done in the face of anxiety experienced by children about the onset of an undesired puberty associated with their assigned sex. We might suggest, then, that being able to 'see' that puberty is 'spread out through a few months' is a relative luxury experienced by parents who do not personally experience dysphoria. Both Kristina and her husband Marc provide further warrant to the idea of taking time, through reference to the idea that someone seen as 'so young' has to make a decision about fertility preservation. For Kristina, ultimately the decision was her daughter's to make, yet this according of agency to Mariah sits in the context of Kristina's own perceptions about the passage of time, and her own non-trans understanding of temporality.

Other parents commented on temporality as a state of being in flux, one that is differentially felt across generations and contexts:

> AMANDA (PARENT OF ASHLEIGH, AGE 15): So they said to Ashleigh would she be prepared to go off blockers for a period of time, partly for fertility so they can collect a sample. And I was sort of saying well, going off blockers will be really bad for her mental health, it will be very stressful. Like I don't want to sound like I'm criticising, but I sort of feel like things are changing rapidly and the kids are here and they're having this treatment but then there's knock on – you know, now you've got this whole

population of kids who started blockers really early, so how do they deal with that? And then, you know, because previously I guess if it was older people transitioning, that's different again, you know, people who've been through one puberty or they might already have children or – you know what I mean? So it seems like … I feel like it's like a crunch point possibly just right now that will clear itself.

In this extract Amanda speaks to the theme of temporality in multiple ways. In the first instance, Amanda's daughter was asked if she wanted to cease puberty blockers 'for a period of time' so as to facilitate fertility preservation. Here a pause in the present is seen as facilitating an option for the future. As Amanda notes, however, such a pause in the present would likely have consequences in the present, potentially overriding any benefit in the future. Amanda then goes on to draw a distinction between differing cohorts of trans people, for some of whom issues of fertility preservation may have been moot, or may have created a different burden. In contrast, for young people like Amanda's daughter, there is a 'crunch point' where a decision has to be made in the context of 'rapid change', with no clear idea of what that might mean for the future.

Fertility preservation and an imagined future

As we introduced in the previous theme, fertility preservation for trans young people in many ways evokes a sense of temporality, one in which young people and their parents are invited to invest in an imagined future, but an imagined future with no fixed or guaranteed outcomes. For some young people, fertility preservation was about creating a possibility, rather than making a firm commitment to a potential future:

> KYA (AGE 17): I just wanted to make sure that [having genetically related children] was going to be an option for me regardless of how I felt at the time. And it's really a thing that's important to me, so I think I wanted to be sure.
>
> JOHANNAH (MOTHER OF KYA): I sort of look at it as an insurance policy. We weren't sure where this would lead at the time we did fertility preservation, we weren't sure that she was going to medically transition. I mean, I think I was 90% sure that you probably would, but I figured it can't hurt to go down that path, and if it turned out that Kya didn't need it, well, it didn't matter, but if it turned out that she did need it then it wouldn't be a hindrance to have done that.

Here Kya refers to fertility preservation as creating an 'option', and her mother Johannah refers to it as an 'insurance policy'. These, however, are quite different accounts. Fertility preservation as an option effectively leaves the door open to a diversity of imagined futures, including having children from stored gametes or not. An insurance policy, by contrast, is typically taken out against the risk of future harm: we take out life insurance to protect our loved ones if we die; we take out home insurance in case we are burgled or our house burns down. So what was Johannah insuring against? Johannah suggests that she was '90% sure' that Kya would medically transition, so it might be that fertility preservation was insurance against the possibility that Kya might commence medical transition and then make a different decision in the future (i.e., accounting for the other '10%'). Alternately, fertility preservation might be an insurance policy against a perceived 'cost' of medical transition: of potentially not being able to have children to whom one is genetically related. While we cannot know for sure from this extract what Johanna meant by the term 'insurance policy', our point here is to highlight potentially differing views on fertility preservation between children and their parents.

Similar to Kya, other young people interviewed were clear that fertility preservation simply created an option:

> INTERVIEWER: And, so, Mariah, what are your thoughts about fertility in the future?
>
> MARIAH (AGE 17): I like the option if I want to have a child in the future. Sometimes, I want a child, I don't want a child, but I'm happy to have that option there.

Other participants too had made decisions about fertility preservation, weighed against an imagined future, and had opted not to preserve their fertility:

> INTERVIEWER: So can you tell me a bit about the discussions about fertility?
>
> ASHLEIGH (AGE 15): Well, I was told that if I didn't go off blockers I wouldn't be able to have a biological baby from myself. And at first I was a bit like – I weighed it all up and honestly, there are other ways – I worked out there are other ways to get a baby but there aren't other ways to get your voice back and stuff. So I just – yeah, I decided that the best option for me was to not worry about that.

For Ashleigh, it would seem, the imagined future she had to negotiate was one in which the potential to have a 'biological baby' remained open, against an accompanying likely future in which undertaking fertility preservation would mean that her voice would change (due to temporarily ceasing puberty blockers) in an undesirable and potentially permanent way. For Ashleigh, and similar to Mariah in the first extract included in this chapter, the possibility of a baby did not constitute enough of a desired imagined future in order to warrant something that was completely undesirable (i.e., voice change).

Conclusions

In this chapter we have explored the topic of fertility preservation for trans young people. Through survey and interview data with parents and young people, we have suggested that there is a tension between the provision of affirming medical care for increasingly younger children, and the potential reproductive rights of such young children. In other words, the provision of affirming medical care brings with it potential challenges in terms of supporting young people to enact their reproductive rights, both in the present and potentially in the future. For some people, this tension results in the suggestion that children are too young to make decisions, and ultimately in the suggestion that affirming medical care should not be given to young children, especially if it might compromise their fertility. Obviously this is not an argument we would support, and it is not an argument that our findings support. Nonetheless, this type of argument is one that needs careful examination in terms of ensuring reproductive justice for trans young people.

One approach to ensuring reproductive justice for trans people is to engage in conversations about reproduction, fertility, and affirming medical care that create a space in which young people can think through the options available to them. As our findings suggest, this includes ensuring that information is available to young people and their parents about reproduction, fertility, and parenting options, and that this is couched in terminology that is inclusive. Examples of this might include using the term 'gametes' rather than sperm or eggs. It might include using conditional language (i.e., 'most girls have a period and can get pregnant, and some people of other genders do too'), rather than definitive exclusionary language.

In our other work focused on sexuality education for trans young people (Riggs & Bartholomaeus, 2018b), we have explored how some young people may re-gender body parts, so as to reduce feelings of dysphoria in the context of intimate encounters. Examples of this might include a trans young man referring to his genitalia as a 'dick', or a 'front hole'. Yet it is rarely the case that sexual health education is inclusive of trans young people (Ferfolja & Ullman, 2021; Shannon, 2016; Shannon & Smith, 2015). Education that is inclusive of all genders, and starting from a young age, provides an opportunity to inform trans young people and their peers about conception, gestation, intimate relationships, and reproductive decision making in ways that are not reliant upon normative gendered assumptions. For example, there would be a place to start this in Australia at a young age, as the National Curriculum includes focus areas in relationships and sexuality as part of Health and Physical Education at Years 3 and 4 (approximately ages 8–10), well before most children would be likely to commence affirming medical care. If trans young people are provided with such information from a young age, it is more likely that by the time they come to the point of having to make decisions about medical treatment, including with regard to fertility preservation, they will be aware and well informed about the options available to them.

Relatedly, it is vitally important that information provided, including in sexual health education, is not itself a conduit for pronatalism. Any information about reproduction or future parenthood must ensure that multiple options are explored in detail, including that not having children is a legitimate and viable option. When discussions do centre on future decisions about children, these should include conception via intercourse, as is currently the norm within such education, but also conception via assisted reproductive technologies, and parenthood via adoption or fostering. Importantly, for all of these pathways to parenthood, potential challenges should be explored with young people. These would include, for example, challenges in conceiving (i.e., potential infertility), challenges associated with assisted reproductive technologies, and the current state of the adoptive and fostering systems. As we noted above, there is no guarantee for trans young people that fertility preservation will result in the conception of a child. This type of information must be available to young people. Similarly, in our research and that of others, as mentioned above, many trans young people emphasise adoption as a potential pathway to future parenthood. Yet, in countries such as Australia, adoption rates are very low, with foster care being the preferred mode of delivering out-of-home care (Riggs & Bartholomaeus, 2016). Providing information about pathways to parenthood through (long-term) foster care, then, is vitally important.

Turning to parents, many parents supported their children in the difficult decisions around medical affirming care and fertility possibilities, and educated themselves on the processes. This was particularly the case in the interviews, where parents who agreed to participate in these dyad interviews may have been more likely to be supportive of their children. However, our findings would also suggest that, for some parents, it is important to provide support services for parents needing to work through potential loss and grief related to their own dreams and assumptions about future grandparenthood, or the normative assumption that their child will ultimately find their life fulfilled by becoming a parent. While these types of assumptions are the product of cultural norms, that does not mean they are any less deeply felt. Providing support services can assist parents in working through feelings that may otherwise serve as a barrier to truly supporting a child to make a decision about fertility preservation. For example, a parent who is strongly invested in becoming a grandparent may strongly encourage, or even insist on a child undertaking fertility preservation. A parent who is overly focused on their own needs may fail to recognise how distressing and dysphoria-inducing fertility preservation can be for a young person. Support for parents is thus essential to ensure that, in turn, parents are able to support their children to make informed decisions.

As our findings would also suggest, matters of reproductive justice are also at stake when available services are limited by geographic context. In Australia, for example, in some states a diversity of fertility preservation techniques are available, whilst in other states fewer are available. This is also the case internationally, and is further compounded by whether or not a particular geographic context provides social healthcare or if services are user-pays. In Australia, for example, fertility preservation for young oncology patients is free, but it is user-pays for trans people of all ages. To ensure reproductive justice for trans young people, increased funding for a diversity of fertility preservation options is needed, including medical research to progress options that at present are only experimental. This of course must be accompanied, as outlined above, with education for trans young people about the likely outcomes of fertility preservation. Otherwise there is the potential that fertility preservation makes a promise to young people that may be unfulfilled.

Finally in terms of our findings, it is important to note that most of the interview participants included in this chapter – those who spoke the most about fertility preservation – were trans girls. In many ways this runs counter to the suggestion we made earlier in this paper, namely that cisgenderism and pronatalism in concert may lead to people assigned female at birth being those most clearly targeted for fertility preservation. Indeed, certainly it may be the case that the trans boys we spoke with were resistant to talking about fertility preservation because they were aware of the normative expectation – the motherhood mandate – that they should want to reproduce, and specifically to carry a child.

Beyond this possible reason for why girls were more likely to talk about fertility preservation than were boys, there are other ways of thinking about the intersections of cisgenderism and pronatalism, as this chapter would suggest. First, our other research on fertility preservation has suggested that medical professionals may view fertility preservation for trans girls and women to be 'easier' (Riggs & Bartholomaeus, 2020). Such an account reduces gamete storage to a mechanical action, devoid of psychological cost, and ignorant of dysphoria. It may thus be that our young female participants were especially targeted due to a perception that gamete storage, where possible, would somehow be easier for them. Second, it is also possible that, as young women, there may have been the pronatalist assumption by medical professionals that in the future they will want to be mothers. In some respects this is positive – that trans girls are viewed as future women and mothers – but on the other hand it is less than positive in its assumption of a motherhood mandate for trans girls. Third, and by contrast, it may have been considered a delicate conversation by medical professionals to explicitly state that a trans boy might want to bear children in the future (though that did not stop one of our parent participants making such a statement). While we cannot know for sure if any of these reasons were in play in the conversations that our young participants undertook with fertility specialists, what these reasons (and likely many others) demonstrate, are the complex intersections of cisgenderism and pronatalism, and their implications for reproductive justice for trans young people.

In conclusion, and as this chapter has demonstrated, fertility preservation for trans young people, and reproductive justice more broadly, is in a state of tension. This is a product of ever-changing medical service provision, the lack of service availability and education, financial costs, normative gendered assumptions about gametes, reproduction, and parenthood, and broader societal attitudes towards the rights of trans people. The solution, of course, is not to compromise trans young people's reproductive rights, but nor is it to insist upon a pronatalist logic. Rather, it is to carefully unpack how cisgenderism shapes each area of tension. It is only when cisgenderism has been unravelled from what is and is not possible for trans young people in terms of fertility preservation, that genuine discussions can occur in which informed consent is truly possible. And ultimately this is the ideal goal of reproductive justice approaches to fertility preservation for trans young people: for there to be respect for young people's right to make decisions, including decisions that may prioritise gender-affirming medical care over potential future parenthood. To do otherwise is to reduce decision making to the default presumption that everyone should want to have (genetically related) children, which is itself counter to the aims of reproductive justice, which focuses on the capacity of individuals to make their own decision about how they might exercise their reproductive rights.

References

Adeleye, A. J., Cedars, M. I., Smith, J., & Mok-Lin, E. (2019). Ovarian stimulation for fertility preservation or family building in a cohort of transgender men. *Journal of Assisted Reproduction and Genetics, 36*(10), 2155–2161.

Armuand, G., Dhejne, C., Olofsson, J. I., & Rodriguez-Wallberg, K. A. (2017). Transgender men's experiences of fertility preservation: A qualitative study. *Human Reproduction, 32*(2), 383–390.

Bartholomaeus, C., & Riggs, D. W. (2020). Transgender and non-binary Australians' experiences with healthcare professionals in relation to fertility preservation. *Culture, Health & Sexuality, 22*(2), 129–145.

Bartholomaeus, C., Riggs, D.W., & Pullen Sansfaçon, A. (2021). Expanding and improving trans affirming care in Australia. Experiences with healthcare professionals among transgender young people and their parents. *Health Sociology Review, 30,* 58–71.

Bauer, G., Lawson, M., Gotovac, S., Couch, B., Ducharme, J., Feder, S., … Temple-Newhook, J. (2018). Trans Youth CAN! A new cohort study of medical, family, and social outcomes for trans and nonbinary youth in Canadian clinics. Poster presented at *World Professional Association for Transgender Health*, November 2–6, Buenos Aries, Argentina.

Braun, V., & Clarke, V. (2006). Using thematic analysis in psychology. *Qualitative Research in Psychology, 3*(2), 77–101.

Chen, D., Kyweluk, M. A., Sajwani, A., Gordon, E. J., Johnson, E. K., Finlayson, C. A., & Woodruff, T. K. (2019). Factors affecting fertility decision-making among transgender adolescents and young adults. *LGBT Health, 6*(3), 107–115.

Chen, D., Matson, M., Macapagal, K., Johnson, E. K., Rosoklija, I., Finlayson, C., … Mustanski, B. (2018). Attitudes toward fertility and reproductive health among transgender and gender-nonconforming adolescents. *Journal of Adolescent Health, 63*(1), 62–68.

Chen, D., Simons, L., Johnson, E. K., Lockart, B. A., & Finlayson, C. (2017). Fertility preservation for transgender adolescents. *Journal of Adolescent Health, 61*(1), 120–123.

Chiniara, L. N., Viner, C., Palmert, M., & Bonifacio, H. (2019). Perspectives on fertility preservation and parenthood among transgender youth and their parents. *Archives of Disease in Childhood, 104*(8), 739–744.

Ferfolja, T., & Ullman, J. (2021). Inclusive pedagogies for transgender and gender diverse children: Parents' perspectives on the limits of discourses of bullying and risk in schools. *Pedagogy, Culture & Society,* 1–18.

Handler, T., Hojilla, J. C., Varghese, R., Wellenstein, W., Satre, D. D., & Zaritsky, E. (2019). Trends in referrals to a pediatric transgender clinic. *Pediatrics.* https://doi.org/10.1542/peds.2019-1368

Harris, R. M., Kolaitis, I. N., & Frader, J. E. (2020). Ethical issues involving fertility preservation for transgender youth. *Journal of Assisted Reproduction and Genetics, 37*(10), 2453–2462.

Hsieh, H. F., & Shannon, S. E. (2005). Three approaches to qualitative content analysis. *Qualitative Health Research, 15*(9), 1277–1288.

Kaltiala, R., Bergman, H., Carmichael, P., de Graaf, N. M., Egebjerg Rischel, K., Frisén, L., ... Waehre, A. (2020). Time trends in referrals to child and adolescent gender identity services: A study in four Nordic countries and in the UK. *Nordic Journal of Psychiatry, 74*(1), 40–44.

Kyweluk, M. A., Sajwani, A., & Chen, D. (2018). Freezing for the future: Transgender youth respond to medical fertility preservation. *International Journal of Transgenderism, 19*(4), 401–416.

Nahata, L., Tishelman, A. C., Caltabellotta, N. M., & Quinn, G. P. (2017). Low fertility preservation utilization among transgender youth. *Journal of Adolescent Health, 61*(1), 40–44.

Oliphant, J., Veale, J., Macdonald, J., Carroll, R., Johnson, R., Harte, M., et al. (2018). *Guidelines for gender affirming healthcare for gender diverse and transgender children, young people and adults in Aotearoa*, New Zealand. Transgender Health Research Lab, University of Waikato. Retrieved from https://researchcommons.waikato.ac.nz/handle/10289/12160

Persky, R. W., Gruschow, S. M., Sinaii, N., Carlson, C., Ginsberg, J. P., & Dowshen, N. L. (2020). Attitudes toward fertility preservation among transgender youth and their parents. *Journal of Adolescent Health, 67*(4), 583–589.

Pro-choice Public Education Project and the Lesbian, Gay, Bisexual and Transgender Community Centre. (n.d.). *Silenced bodies: Conversations with gay men, bisexual and transgender persons, and queer women of color on sexual and reproductive health, rights and justice*. Retrieved from https://web.archive.org/web/20130330233944/http://www.gaycenter.org/files/imce/docs/causesSilencedbodies.pdf

Riggs, D. W. (2019). An examination of 'just in case' arguments as they are applied to fertility preservation for transgender people. In V. Mackie, S. Ferber & N. Marks (Eds.), *The reproductive industry: Intimate experiences and global processes* (pp. 69–78). New York: Lexington Books.

Riggs, D. W., & Bartholomaeus, C. (2020). Toward trans reproductive justice: A qualitative analysis of views on fertility preservation for Australian transgender and non-binary people. *Journal of Social Issues, 76*(2), 314–337.

Riggs, D. W., & Bartholomaeus, C. (2018a). Fertility preservation decision making amongst Australian transgender and non-binary adults. *Reproductive Health, 15*(1), 181.

Riggs, D.W., & Bartholomaeus, C. (2018b). Transgender young people's narratives of intimacy and sexual health: Implications for sexuality education. *Sex Education, 18*, 376–390.

Riggs, D. W., & Bartholomaeus, C. (2016). *Australian family diversity: An historical overview 1960–2015*. Adelaide: Flinders University.

Riggs, D. W., Bartholomaeus, C., & Pullen Sansfaçon, A. (2020). 'If they didn't support me, I most likely wouldn't be here': Transgender young people and their parents negotiating medical treatment in Australia. *International Journal of Transgenderism, 21*(1), 3–15.

Shannon, B. (2016). Comprehensive for who? Neoliberal directives in Australian 'comprehensive' sexuality education and the erasure of GLBTIQ identity. *Sex Education, 16*(6), 573–585.

Shannon, B., & Smith, S. J. (2015). 'A lot more to learn than where babies come from': Controversy, language and agenda setting in the framing of school-based sexuality education curricula in Australia. *Sex Education, 15*(6), 641–654.

Telfer, M., Tollit, M., & Feldman, D. (2015). Transformation of health-care and legal systems for the transgender population. *Journal of Paediatrics and Child Health, 51*(11), 1051–1053.

Telfer, M., Tollit, M., Pace, C., & Pang, K. (2017). *Australian Standards of Care and Treatment Guidelines: For trans and gender diverse children and adolescents.* Melbourne: The Royal Children's Hospital.

World Professional Association for Transgender Health. (2011). *Standards of care for the health of transsexual, transgender, and gender nonconforming people,* 7th version. Retrieved from www.wpath.org/publications/soc

9

YOUNG MEN, TRANS/MASCULINE, AND NON-BINARY PEOPLE'S VIEWS ABOUT PREGNANCY

Damien W. Riggs, Carla A. Pfeffer, Francis Ray White, Sally Hines and Ruth Pearce

Introduction

Over the past three decades there has been a shift in thinking about fathers, moving beyond the normative ideal of the traditional 'breadwinner' (Hunter & Riggs, 2020). Associated with this shift has been increased attention to how cisgender young men conceptualize a future in which they may become fathers (Marsiglio, Hutchinson, & Cohan, 2000; Bartholomaeus & Riggs, 2020; Thompson & Lee, 2011; Thompson, Lee, & Adams, 2013). Much of the literature in this area suggests that young cisgender men envisage future fatherhood as an opportunity for growth (i.e., in terms of self-understanding), a time for connection (i.e., developing a loving bond with a child), and as markedly different from their own experiences of being fathered (i.e., wanting to be involved with their children, rather than primarily fulfilling a traditional breadwinner role). The literature on first time heterosexual cisgender fathers, however, suggests that some of the imagined futures that young men hold may not always come to fruition, particularly with regard to the equal distribution of household labour (Riggs & Bartholomaeus, 2020a).

One reason for potential discrepancies between imagined and actual fatherhood among young heterosexual cisgender men pertains to the relationship between ideals and ideologies. A young heterosexual cisgender man may hold the ideal of equal parenting, or the ideal that they will be closely involved with, and connected to, their child's life. Yet normative ideologies about parenting, and gendered ideologies in particular, may shape whether or not such ideals actually occur in practice. The discrepancy between ideals and ideologies is perhaps most evident with regard to essentialist arguments about gender and parenting. Research suggests that while some young heterosexual cisgender men may hold liberal views about their role as fathers in their children's lives, this may be paired with essentialist beliefs about gender (Edley & Wetherell, 1999). For example, young men may appreciate that

DOI: 10.4324/9781003138310-9

gender imbalances in terms of household labour are both unjust and a potential threat to relationship happiness. But at the same time, they may hold the view that women are 'naturally' designed to raise children. Here essentialist views collapse the capacity to bear a child, with the capacity to raise a child, positioning women as inherently predisposed to undertaking a primary caregiving role.

Wrapped up in essentialist beliefs about parenting are young cisgender men's negotiations with discourses of masculinity. Again, many young heterosexual cisgender men may seek to challenge the traditional breadwinner role when it comes to fatherhood, but they must do so in a broader social context where caregiving is normatively associated with femininity, and paid work outside the home normatively associated with masculinity (Hunter & Riggs, 2020). Obviously, such essentialist beliefs are open to change, but for many people change requires active and purposive resistance to enshrined beliefs. In the context of fatherhood, and particularly first-time fatherhood, young men may struggle to reconcile the desire to enact change with the heightened demands of new fatherhood, and may default to culturally prescribed norms related to parenting roles. Such norms impact men who do seek to challenge normative gender roles and expectations, who are often met with sanctions from others with regard to their masculinity and parenting role, whereby both enacting involved fathering and adopting a normative place within discourses of masculinity may be heavily regulated by others (Hunter & Riggs, 2020).

Importantly, essentialist beliefs about parenting have negative impacts not solely for cisgender young men. Extensive attention has been paid to how essentialist beliefs about parenting fundamentally shape cisgender women's experiences (Pascoe Leahy & Bueskens, 2019). This includes the assumption that cisgender women should uniformly desire to have children, that they should uniformly find happiness in mothering, and that cisgender women automatically know what to do when it comes to parenting. Such assumptions marginalize the experiences of cisgender women who do not want to have children as well as those who are unable to have children. They also serve to discredit the experiences of women who feel regret about having children, or who find it difficult to bond with their children. And they can often translate into cisgender women being provided with inadequate parental support, under the assumption that gestation automatically equates with adequate knowledge about how to raise children.

Often missing from these important areas of focus on heterosexual cisgender men and women, however, has been attention to other groups of people for whom plans about future parenthood, the injunction to parenthood, and recognition as potential future parents are often left unsaid. In this chapter we focus specifically on young men, trans/masculine, and non-binary people. We use the term 'young men, trans/masculine, and non-binary people' to refer to people who were assigned female at birth, but report their identity as, for example, male, man, trans, masculine, transmasculine, non-binary, genderqueer, or agender. While a growing body of research has focused on the pregnancy-related experiences of this diverse group of people (e.g., Charter et al., 2018; Hoffkling et al., 2017; Light et al., 2014), less often has attention been paid to how young men, trans/masculine, and non-binary people think about pregnancy in general, and how they think about potential pregnancy for themselves into the future. Drawing on focus groups conducted with 18 young men, trans/masculine, and non-binary people across three countries, in this chapter we argue that essentialist beliefs about reproduction very much impact the experiences of this diverse group of young people. In the sections that follow we first provide an overview of the limited body of literature in this area. We then briefly describe the background to our project, before presenting the findings of our thematic analysis of the focus group data. We conclude the chapter by exploring what our findings mean for a trans reproductive justice approach.

Literature overview and project background

As outlined in the first chapter of this book, cisgenderism as an ideology shapes and potentially limits the ways in which trans people are able to enact reproductive and sexual rights. Importantly, and as the following examples highlight, cisgenderism – through its emphasis on assuming a normative relationship between assigned sex and gender – enables what would otherwise be a contradictory set of ideological claims to be rhetorically reconciled. Consider, for example, the long-standing position, now increasingly referred to as trans-exclusionary radical feminism, in which transgender women are viewed as usurping the place of cisgender women (Vincent, Erikainen, & Pearce, 2020). At least part of this argument relies upon essentialist arguments about what constitutes a woman, emphasizing the capacity to gestate as key. Yet ignored in this type of argument is the fact that many cisgender women cannot or do not want to bear a child. Such accounts of transgender women sit in a broader context of particular radical feminist arguments about the function of patriarchy in usurping the role of (nominally cisgender) women in reproduction, particularly with regard to assisted reproductive technologies being framed as an inherently masculinist enterprise, one that ultimately is seen as denying what is viewed as the fundamental role of cisgender women in societies as those who reproduce (Corea, 1985).

Such expressed concerns about women and reproduction have arguably reached their zenith in public discourse about men and pregnancy. In one turn, public discourse about trans men and pregnancy has often adopted an essentialist approach, denying that trans men are men. In another turn, trans men who undertake a pregnancy are positioned as men whose pregnancies further usurp the role of women as reproducers. In yet another turn, trans men are positioned as 'naturally fulfilling a biological destiny', drawing on normative assumptions about people assigned female at birth and reproduction. In the latter such account trans men are both tentatively recognized as men, but also tied to bodies that are positioned by others as female. Such bodies are thus subjected to the same pronatalist injunctions as are other bodies read as female (Riggs & Bartholomaeus, 2019b). Meanwhile, trans people who undertake a pregnancy but do *not* identify as men (such as transmasculine non-binary individuals, for example) are typically erased from the conversation entirely. Cisgenderism, then, while unified by a set of normative assumptions, takes many forms that negatively impact upon how trans people's reproductive decisions are both understood and enacted.

As one of the most well-known men who has undertaken pregnancies, considerable academic attention has been paid to the life of Thomas Beatie. The findings of academic research very much mirror the contradictory accounts outlined above. For example, Landau (2012) interviewed a group of North American cisgender women of 'child-bearing age', and asked them to respond to two images of Beatie that were widely circulated in the public: one of Beatie holding his pregnant stomach, and one of the cover of Beatie's book that featured both Beatie and his then wife holding his pregnant stomach. Of the women interviewed, most viewed the first image as inherently masculine, noting Beatie's body and facial hair, his large hands, and dismissing his pregnancy stomach as a 'beer belly'. Some women were critical of the image, suggesting that 'even as a joke' it served to usurp the role of women as reproducers. When presented with the second image, however, some of the women revised their account of Beatie, which had previously marked him as a man. Instead, some of the women remarked on the scars on his chest (a result of chest surgery), making conjectures about his gender history, revising their gendering of Beatie (from all initially referring to Beatie as 'he', to some questioning or changing the pronouns they used), and questioning more broadly the ethics and medical possibilities of trans men bearing children.

Riggs (2014) has examined the interview that Beatie and his then wife undertook with Oprah Winfrey. As Riggs argues, Winfrey repeatedly invited Beatie to explain to the audience how it was that he could be a pregnant man. This included asking Beatie to share his experiences with regard to the death of his mother (with Winfrey suggesting that the death of Beatie's mother meant he had 'no feminine images'), Winfrey repeatedly contradicting Beatie's account of his masculinity (which he framed as a lifelong feeling, and Winfrey countered this with a focus on Beatie taking part in Miss Teen Hawaii), and Winfrey insisting on a prurient focus on Beatie's genitalia. Throughout the interview Winfrey emphasized a highly normative account of gender, drawing on cisgenderist ideologies to suggest that pregnancy is the same for people of all genders, that there are only two genders, and reinforcing a normative account of Beatie's reproductive and sexed body. Throughout the interview Beatie effectively countered Winfrey's line of argument, yet in so doing was repeatedly forced to adopt a relatively normative account of his gender as masculine.

The topic of negotiations with masculinity are replete across the literature on men, trans/masculine, and non-binary people and pregnancy. Riggs (2013), for example, has explored how trans men, in their public self-representations, account for masculinity as part of their pregnancy journeys. For some men, their masculinity is positioned as tenuous in the face of highly feminized narratives of pregnancy. More specifically, their masculinity is positioned as tenuous by *other people*: by people who misgender them in hospitals, by strangers who refuse to view them as pregnant men, and by broader discourses that position all pregnancies as by default undertaken by women. Other men may feel within themselves that pregnancy compromises their masculinity, particularly with regard to inhabiting a pregnant body that they struggle to view as masculine. Yet other men may refuse the feminization of pregnancy, instead seeing their pregnant or lactating bodies as serving a purpose, one that does not inherently undermine their experience of their masculinity. Indeed, in an account of their own pregnancy, Wallace (2010) talks about the 'manly art of pregnancy', noting that a

> pregnant person is at once a biologist, a mechanic, a weight lifter, and someone providing for hir family. Women can do those things, of course, but our culture still views them as masculine things, and in this way pregnancy made me more of a man, not less of one … Pregnancy helped me look, feel and act more like an archetype of Man, and eventually lifted me to its pinnacle by making me a dad.
>
> *(p. 133)*

In other research too, men, trans/masculine, and non-binary people have positioned pregnancy as an opportunity to enact a new understanding of gender and of the self. Non-binary or genderqueer gestational parents interviewed as part of a study by Carpenter and Niesen (2021), for example, saw pregnancy as an opportunity to create a 'queer experience' of reproduction. Similarly, in Tasker and Gato's (2020) focus group research with 11 trans or non-binary people (of whom four were men and five were non-binary), many of the participants spoke about a desire to have a child in the future, even in the face of experiences of, or presumptions about the likelihood of, cisgenderism within reproductive services. Participants were particularly focused on the importance of needing a diversity of forms of support, eschewing the normative assumption that having a child can only occur in the context of a couple relationship. Interviews undertaken by Ryan (2009) with ten trans men also highlighted that many of the participants saw parenting as an opportunity to rework entrenched norms about 'patriarchal fatherhood', holding up their diverse experiences of gender as offering the potential to enable new ways of thinking about what it means to raise children. Fischer (2021) too found from interviews with ten non-binary gestational parents that many valued having the space in which to engage in parenting that resisted traditional gender norms.

The data we explore in this chapter are drawn from a broader international study focused on men, trans/masculine, and non-binary people's experiences of reproduction. The study more broadly has involved interviews with this diverse group of people, focusing on their experiences of pregnancy (see Riggs et al., 2021 for more information about the broader project). In the study, however, we were also interested to explore how young men, trans/masculine, and non-binary people who had not undertaken a pregnancy viewed pregnancy for trans people. To that end, we ran focus groups to explore some of the topics introduced above in our overview of the literature, specifically in terms of views about pregnancy and masculinity, views about public representations of men, trans/masculine and non-binary people and pregnancy, and the factors that shape people's decisions about possible future pregnancies. Our participants were 18 young men, trans/masculine, or non-binary people who attended one of five focus groups. Two focus groups were held in Australia, two in the United States, and one in the United Kingdom. Three of the focus groups were convened face to face, and two were held online. Participants were recruited via posts on social media, including to groups specifically for trans people. In the United Kingdom, the focus group was held in collaboration with a not-for-profit organization that specializes in providing support to trans young people.

Of the 18 participants, the average age was 23 years. In terms of gender, eight participants reported their gender as non-binary, five as trans men, two as agender, two as transmasculine and one as genderfluid. In terms of ethnicity, 16 of the participants reported their ethnicity as white/Caucasian/English/British, one as Asian, and one as mixed race. In terms of sexuality, six participants reported their sexuality as queer, six as bisexual, four as pansexual, one as asexual, and one as demisexual. When it came to analysing the data, we read through all of the focus group transcripts as one corpus of data. While we acknowledge that this has the potential to marginalize regional differences – and certainly in future publications we intend to focus more closely on any such differences – for the present chapter we sought to provide a broad overview of the most common ways that our focus group participants spoke about pregnancy. Adopting a thematic analytic approach (Braun & Clarke, 2006), the first author developed themes from the full data corpus, and identified indicative extracts for each theme. These are presented below along with analysis of the extracts at both the latent and semantic level.

Themes developed from focus groups

Pronatalism directed towards men, trans/masculine, and non-binary people

In this first theme, focus group participants spoke about experiencing an injunction from other people to reproduce, or at the very least to view the loss of the capacity to reproduce (as a result of, for example, a hysterectomy or commencing hormone therapy) as a significant issue. As was explored in the first chapter of this book, trans reproductive justice encompasses not simply the right to have children and raise them safely, but also the right to *not* have children, which included the rights not to be compelled to reproduce. As has been found in other research (e.g., Riggs & Bartholomaeus, 2020b), some of our focus group participants spoke about experiencing pressure from family members to have children, as is evident in the following extract:

> ASH: People see us as people getting rid of their ability to give life, but some trans men don't give up that part of their bodies. So it just really depends on, like, who they are really.

OLLIE: Well I've never actually heard that … like, that people see, like, trans men or transmasculine people as, like, giving up their ability to give life. I feel, like, that's really intense.

ASH: That's really what my mother said to me. Because my sister is asexual so she doesn't do sex. So my mum told me I was her only chance of having grandbabies. And then she found out I was trans and I was getting that cut out. And she got mad.

For Ash, his mother placed her expectations about having a grandchild onto him, and in so doing effectively reduced his body to a body capable of gestation. Rather than supporting the decisions that Ash made with regard to his body (i.e., in terms of having a hysterectomy), his mother 'got mad', precisely because his decision ran counter to his mother's desire for grandchildren. Certainly, from the extract above we cannot know if his mother was more broadly affirming of him as a man, but certainly in the extract above we can see that the reduction of Ash to a body capable of gestation does not inherently affirm his experience of what it means to be a man. Obviously, as our project more broadly shows, for some men, trans/masculine, and non-binary people gestational parenthood is very much an aspect of their experience of their gender and embodiment. But for people such as Ash, this was not his desire, yet he was nonetheless subjected to the views of his mother on the topic.

For other focus group participants, pronatalist assumptions were voiced by healthcare professionals, such as in the following extract:

DAVID: Um, I know when I started testosterone, like, they asked me very extensively about if I would ever want to have kids. And to be able to get testosterone, I had to tell them that I probably would never carry and that I was okay with possibly being sterile. Because I am, I mean, it's not something that I feel strongly for, strongly negative about. Um, but I know a lot of, like, cis women have a very hard time trying to get hysterectomies. Um, I had a friend, she's twenty-seven now and she doesn't want to have children. And she had to go to eight doctors to be able to get a hysterectomy, a lot of them asked what her boyfriend thought about that and, you know, that kind of stuff. So I can see it being as hard for trans people, especially trans men. People still have the stigma of, oh, you might want to have kids in the future, or maybe you want to do something, er, with your eggs, maybe you want to freeze them.

It is of course important, in order to ensure the reproductive rights of men, trans/masculine, and non-binary people, that healthcare professionals address the topic of reproduction prior to decision making about gender affirming medical treatment. Yet, as this extract would suggest, there is a difference between addressing the topic and outlining options, and making it a requirement that people are certain about their future decisions. As is true for any person, trans people have the right to change their mind, and for men, trans/masculine, and non-binary people this might include deciding to commence hormone therapy, and later deciding to cease treatment for a period of time in order to potentially undertake a pregnancy. As David suggests, this type of logic about certainty is equally used to question the decisions made by cisgender women who seek a hysterectomy at a young age. Inherent in this type of questioning, and similar to the questioning that David suggests in terms of trans men possibly wanting children in the future, is pronatalism: that all people should, or at least are likely to, want to have children in the future, and that this is especially true for those who are capable of gestation.

Turning point in decision making about future parenthood

Given the broader context of pronatalism, as we explored in the previous theme, and how pronatalism intersects with cisgenderism (such as the normative expectation that people with bodies that can gestate will undertake a pregnancy), some of our focus group participants spoke about having to make mindful decisions about reproduction, decisions that required developing a critical take on gendered norms about reproduction. One focus group participant noted, for example, how critical reflection enabled them to realize that they don't want to bear a child:

> OLLIE: When I got in to my undergrad, I was still at that point identifying as, like, a straight woman actually. And, um, dated a trans guy. Um, and he was adopted and so, like, adoption to him was super important. And so, like, at that point, like, I was, like, oh I don't have to ... like, I don't have to be pregnant if I want to have children. I don't know. Like, something clicked in that moment and I was like, oh, like, I don't have to do that. Um, and then from that moment on I was like, yeah, like, that just doesn't seem like something I would do. And, like, I don't have to, so that's cool.

As Ollie suggests, they experienced a 'click in that moment', where they came to realize that simply because, at that time, they identified as a 'straight woman', this did not automatically mean that they should want to be pregnant. For Ollie, this was part of a broader shift to understanding that not only was pregnancy not something they wanted, but the gendered box to which they had been assigned was also not something that reflected their own experience. In the following extract, PJ too talks about how normative boxes shaped their coming to a place of understanding about pregnancy.

> PJ: With the whole boxing it into being a female, I think I put more pressure on myself to box myself out of that and not take into consideration what I actually want in terms of myself and ignoring gender as a box. 'Cause whether I do or don't, it's not to do with gender, it's to do with the fact of how I see my life going in a direction, hopefully. That's good in life. So I also went from being in the gender clinic basically saying, "I do not want

children, keep them away from me". I don't want to be part of a child biologically because that would mean I was accepting that I'm female. But I've sort of had a complete 180. And now I'm at a point where I do want to have children, not only biologically, but I do want to carry them.

KITE: Yeah, with the stigma of it being so gendered, especially with the nature of getting any gender confirmation stuff. You have to be so sure, and you have to have lived as your gender for two years. What even is that? So there's a tendency to force yourself into the mindset of being like, "No I don't want anything remotely female in my life, nothing, nothing, nothing. I don't even want to have kids at all, too female, go away!" When actually, yeah, it's something that if you stand back a second, you're like, "Actually it's not a gendered thing".

Different to Ollie, PJ suggests that their turning point was from not wanting to be pregnant, to wanting to carry a child. This '180', as PJ describes it, required PJ to critically unpack the normative assumption that 'female' and 'pregnancy' constituted the same box. For PJ, instead, pregnancy is 'not to do with gender', and thus a decision to potentially bear a child in the future was not a reflection of PJ's gender. Kite in turn reflected PJ's comments, noting that there is a 'stigma' associated with pregnancy for men, trans/masculine, and non-binary people, given the normative gendered association of pregnancy with womanhood. By contrast, Kite emphasizes that it is possible to resist the 'mindset' that pregnancy = female, and to instead recognize that pregnancy is 'actually not a gendered thing'. We would take Kite here to mean not that pregnancy is not gendered: clearly, as all of the themes in this chapter note, pregnancy is heavily gendered as a result of normative social expectations. Rather, we would read Kite as suggesting that pregnancy doesn't have to be *normatively* gendered: that it does not inherently reflect something about a person's gender.

Prurient focus on trans conception

For some focus group participants, deciding that they would be open to undertaking a pregnancy in the future was not without its concerns. In this theme in particular, participants spoke about the concern that other people's awareness about a potential future pregnancy would be seen as inviting prurient attention to their bodies. As we noted earlier in this chapter, certainly much of the attention given to Thomas Beatie involved a prurient focus on his body (Riggs, 2013). This is reflective of a broader social discourse evident particularly in the media, where trans people's bodies are seen as deserving of, and indeed requiring, public commentary. For participants such as Ollie, a potential future pregnancy was thus fraught by the potential for prurient responses:

OLLIE: And another thing I was thinking about was, I feel like I've seen a lot of, like, representations of, like, um, couples where both partners are trans. And, um ... or, like, a trans man, a trans woman, or a transmasculine person and a trans feminine person. And, like, there's this idea of, like, and they can still get pregnant, like, naturally ... air quotes, air quotes. And, like, this weird, like, fetishization of, like, these, like ... like, assigned sexes still, like, being together and being able to, like, create, like, a natural pregnancy, which is ... I think is, like ... like, a weird representation around, like, trans pregnancy.

In our interviews with men, trans/masculine, and non-binary people who had undertaken a pregnancy, some made recourse to normative language about conception, such as describing conceiving by 'bumpin' uglies', by 'the old-fashioned way', or by 'the conventional way' (Riggs et al., 2021). In so doing, our interview participants reworked the normative assumption that reproductive intercourse inherently reflects heterosexual intercourse, which was especially true for our non-heterosexual participants who were in relationships with cisgender men. While these examples from our interview participants demonstrate that it is possible to reclaim or rework normative understandings of conception, for focus group participants such as Ollie the idea of conception evoked the potential for 'fetishization', referring specifically to a prurient focus on bodies normatively associated with assigned sex. Parker explicitly noted that he wouldn't want to be pregnant precisely because of the potential for a prurient focus on his body:

> PARKER: Like actually, the more I think about this, it's like ... like, I guess some of the tangible reasons why I wouldn't want to personally be pregnant is that, like, when I think about, like, the very fragile understanding of my gender that my, like, colleagues have who, like, I am out to, like, yes, they recognize me as male and, like, no, they didn't watch me transition. But I am willing to bet that if I showed up to work pregnant, their gears would probably start turning in their head ... like, there's this Internet meme going around right now that's, like, when a couple says they're trying to conceive, like, what ... what I actually hear them saying is that they've been, like, you know, going at it with no protection or whatever. And, like, if you extend that to a trans person, it's like, okay, like, what I'm saying is like, I am a man who is pregnant. And what my colleagues are hearing is that, like, okay, undressing that person in my head and have come to the terms that they have a vagina or like, has a uterus and ovaries. And, like, even the, like, concept of that is something that makes me, like ... even though it's like not even something I could, like, literally do, even the idea of, like, the thought experiment makes me, like, viscerally uncomfortable.

For Parker, becoming pregnant may be seen as an invitation to others to conjecture about his body, an invitation that reflects a broader cultural obsession with trans people's bodies. In one respect, then, for Parker pregnancy potentially removes any presumption of embodied privacy, instead, in effect, making one's body visible to a cultural imaginary that makes a series of normative assumptions about the configuration of the bodies involved in conception. Parker's points speak to a very specific form of reproductive justice, namely the right to privacy about one's body and one's reproductive practices. Again, the broader cultural obsession with trans people's bodies in effect denies any right to reproductive privacy.

Pregnancy and negotiations with assumptions about masculinity

As we noted earlier in this chapter, pregnancy can bring with it a diversity of views about masculinity for men, trans/masculine, and non-binary people. For some people, undertaking a pregnancy can be experienced as undermining one's sense of one's masculinity, either due to the views of others, or due to one's own embodied experiences of pregnancy (which are certainly not separate from broader cisgenderist narratives that equate pregnancy with womanhood). For other people, by contrast, pregnancy is viewed as a masculine enterprise. Both of these positions were evident in our focus groups. In terms of pregnancy undermining masculinity, some participants endorsed this viewpoint:

> ASH: I feel, like, being pregnant takes a lot away from masculinity. But getting someone pregnant gives you so much masculinity. Like, if you think about it … 'cause they have the ways where it's, like … you can use someone else's sperm and you can, like, use something and then you got her pregnant. But, like … I don't know. I'm sure, like, being pregnant would take away from the whole idea of 'I'm a man'. Like, I see men who, like … trans men who get pregnant and I'm like, go you, and I'll support it. But me personally, I can never get pregnant.

In this extract, while Ash is supportive of men who undertake a pregnancy, for him there is still a strong sense in which masculinity is inherently associated with 'getting someone pregnant'. Here Ash evokes a normative understanding of masculinity, echoing what might broadly be referred to as hegemonic masculinity (Connell & Messerschmidt, 2005), one in which men are seen as agentic, and women by contrast are seen as passive recipients (i.e., 'you got her pregnant'). Other participants too implicitly acknowledged the effects of discourses of hegemonic masculinity on their thinking about men and pregnancy:

> Lee: I think logically I want to say pregnancy can be a masculine thing, but annoyingly my subconscious was immediately like, I don't associate that. Which I think is that sort of stuff that's ingrained in you, that even when you're a part of this community it's sometimes a conscious thing to sort of fight against. So … I guess that is in the back of my mind, so it's probably going to be in the back of a lot of people's, which is an issue.

As has been raised in critiques of the concept of hegemonic masculinity (e.g., Connell & Messerschmidt, 2005), the concept refers less to the actual experiences or practices of all men, and more to a collective imaginary about what constitutes a normative masculinity, or as Lee suggests, a 'subconscious' understanding, one that is 'ingrained in you'. As such, for participants like Lee and Ash, there was a tension between respecting the reproductive decisions of trans men, and having a perception about cultural norms of masculinity.

By contrast, other focus group participants actively endorsed the idea that pregnancy could be a masculine enterprise, with some participants acknowledging that a refusal to see pregnancy as masculine constituted a form of 'toxic masculinity':

> JIM: I definitely think [pregnancy] could be [masculine]. I know I … I see a lot of, like, news stories about, oh, this trans man carried, er, the child for the relationship, 'cause whatever reason here. And those articles are really cool and I've never thought of them as being less a man or anything. And toxic masculinity is a hell of a problem. I don't know, I just think it definitely could be a masculine thing because pregnancy is, like, a really difficult and hard thing.

Jim's comments here in many ways echo Wallace (2010), who suggests that pregnancy can be a 'manly art' because it evokes normative concepts of masculinity, with Jim specifically suggesting that it is 'really difficult and hard'. This type of account of pregnancy as masculine draws attention to some of the problems associated with framing pregnancy as masculine. Given the types of normative associations attached to the concept of masculinity – associations that are often sexist or patriarchal – it is difficult to speak of 'masculine pregnancy' without resorting to traditionally masculinist discourses. Other participants too equated pregnancy with masculinity through recourse to normative assumptions about men's bodies:

> PARKER: Um, and so when I think about, um, like masculinity and pregnancy, for me it's like, okay, like I've had top surgery, like, if I, you know, magically had a uterus and was able to get pregnant, um, like I don't think it would necessarily change my sense of masculinity because, like, with the way I look, like … I mean, I'm a little bit heavy set, like if I ate a lot of food, like … I mean, like, I might be, like, bloated to the point where it looked like I had a baby bump, or something like that. So, like, having that, like, you know, like beer … beer gut or whatever, doesn't change my sense of masculinity, it almost of kind of, in a funny way, it makes me feel like, oh, like, I'm a man's man, with, like a [laugh] a little bit of, like, a beer stomach going on.

Echoing Landau's (2012) interviews with cisgender women, here Parker suggests that, if anything, being pregnant would make him 'a man's man', as it could appear that he has a 'beer gut'. Similar to Jim, then, Parker suggests that pregnancy can be a masculine enterprise precisely because it changes trans men's bodies in ways that make them potentially appear as readable as (cisgender) men. This, of course, is a problematic account of masculinity for trans men, as it requires adherence to a particular bodily norm, one that may not be appealing to all trans men, and one that more broadly reinforces cisgenderist and normatively masculinist understanding of trans men's bodies. Normatively masculinist accounts of men were again evident in other participants' accounts of pregnancy:

> JAKE: I mean I don't really see why there's any reason that [pregnancy] couldn't be [masculine]. There's a lot of things about it that are pretty hard core and would be associated with traditional masculine traits, such as pushing a whole human out of your genitals, or being sliced open so that a whole human can be removed from your body. That's pretty intense, it's very extreme. So those traditional qualities of masculinity could definitely be applied to it, I think.

Here again, normative accounts of masculinity as 'hard core', 'intense', or 'extreme' are positioned as applicable to pregnancy among men, trans/masculine, and non-binary people. The challenge in this type of masculinist account, however, is that it raises questions about its applicability to pregnancy in general (i.e., in framing 'hard core', 'intense', or 'extreme' as masculine attributes, there is a denial that cisgender women, for example, experience pregnancy as 'hard core', 'intense', or 'extreme'), which has particular implications for men, trans/masculine, and non-binary people who undertake a pregnancy and who do not identify as masculine, as the following participant elaborated:

> KARL: I just think whether you would associate pregnancy with masculinity is super subjective. If I were pregnant I wouldn't associate it with masculinity but that's because I don't identify as masculine. For me, it wouldn't be an experience of masculinity, but if you do identify as transmasculine and you are pregnant, then kind of inherently it is masculine, right? Because it's a part of your experience and it is, whether you want it to be or not, it's inherently gendered. So yeah. I think it's really subjective whether that's true for you, or not.

Karl makes two important points. First, that whether or not pregnancy is experienced as masculine is dependent on your own experience of your gender. This is an important counter to the assumption that all men, trans/masculine, or non-binary people experience their gender as masculine. Rather than the only options for experiencing gender as being limited to masculine or feminine, Karl signals that there are other ways of experiencing gender, and further, that there is no normative association between one's gender and one's experience of it. Second, Karl makes the point that pregnancy is not masculine because of particular actions, as suggested by some of the previous participants. Rather, pregnancy can be masculine precisely because a person experiences their gender as masculine.

Pregnant men as a problem for trans communities

In many ways, the views about pregnancy and masculinity that we explored in the previous theme directly relate to the views included in this final theme, specifically with regard to the idea that there are specific ideals that some people hold about what it means to be trans or gender diverse, and men, trans/masculine, and non-binary people who undertake a pregnancy are seen as failing these ideals. As was outlined in the first chapter of this book, the concept of transnormativity refers to the assumption that that there is only one way of being trans or gender diverse. While the first chapter of this book explored how transnormativity is directed towards trans people by cisgender people, including medical professionals, in this final theme we explore evocations of transnormativity within trans communities. Importantly, the participants included in this theme did not endorse transnormativity, but rather spoke about how it occurs with regard to pregnancy, as we can see in the following extract:

> PARKER: In these [social media] groups, like, a lot of trans men who, like, post about pregnancy or, like, post links to, like, these, like, viral stories about 'trans man gets pregnant', or like Instagram accounts, they get, like, totally raked over the coals by, like, a lot of the posters in the group who are just, like, this is a shame to our community and people are gonna be confused and think that, like, trans men want to have babies and that's disgusting, and, like, that makes you a woman, like why would you even want to be a man if you would do that.

In this extract, Parker talks about tension within trans social media groups, tensions that arise in regard to transnormative views about trans men and pregnancy. As Parker notes, pregnant men are viewed by some people as 'shameful', as they may 'confuse' other (cisgender) people who already struggle to understand and accept trans people. Here there is a sense in which trans people are expected to pander to the broader cisgender population in order to warrant inclusion: to not do anything that could cause 'confusion'. Other participants specifically noted that in some sectors of trans communities, pregnancy is seen as inherently feminine, meaning that pregnancy should be avoided for any man, trans/masculine, or non-binary person:

> ROSA: It's really weird, because I have these two dichotomous communities. I have one friend who's also non-binary and they would like, they constantly talk about having kids and how their mum's been real inspirational about wanting to raise someone. Have sort of that really nice, close relationship. And I have others that have literally the same sort of sentiments that have been brought up, like, "You're not trans if you want to get pregnant, you're not, you're like, if you're designated female at birth don't even transition if you think about anything feminine", it is a really weird dichotomy.

As Rosa notes, there is an interesting dichotomy in their experience between a friend feeling affirmed to potentially have children in the future, including by a supportive mother, and community members who suggest that men, trans/masculine, and non-binary people who have undertaken a pregnancy are not actually trans. Given that it is often the opposite – as we found in our interview research, where for some men, trans/masculine, and non-binary people trans communities were supportive while families were not – it is interesting to note here the perception that sometimes it is communities who can endorse and enforce transnormative understandings. In the final extract below Jake makes some important points about the mismatch between trans reproductive justice and transnormativity in trans communities:

> JAKE: Well some people in the trans community are super against people being pregnant which I find weird. Because I feel like if it's not your body then you don't really have a say about whether someone's pregnant or not. Whether they are pregnant or not, or whether someone is trans and is pregnant, it doesn't affect you, so it kind of frustrates me because there's so much control over trans people's bodies and ability to access different transitional medical care. There's so much that you have to go through to access those things. Or when people say, "Oh, you shouldn't be pregnant if you're trans because you're not really trans if you become pregnant" it really makes me angry because if people choose to do that, it's almost as if they are trying to control other people in the same way that they have been controlled. I think that is very messed up.

As Jake notes, "if it's not your body then you don't really have a say". Yet as they also note, some trans people seem to want to enact transnormative control in ways similar to that which they would have experienced within medical care. Whether such views are about staking a claim to a place within the norm, or about the wholesale acceptance of transnormative discourses within the medical professions, cannot be determined on the basis of this extract. But what Jake points to is a wider phenomenon in which cisgenderism as an ideology is not limited to cisgender people: it can influence the views that trans people hold with regard to pregnancy, and which they can attempt to enforce upon others to the detriment of individual reproductive autonomy.

Conclusions

We started this chapter by considering the views of cisgender younger men with regard to future fatherhood, highlighting that there are tensions between the desire to enact fatherhood beyond the norm of the 'traditional breadwinner', and the impact of normative gendered assumptions. Research on trans people who are, or who desire to be, gestational parents similarly highlights tensions, specifically with regard to the desire to enact parenthood in ways that refuse gendered stereotypes, and the impact of cisgenderism in terms of how trans gestational parents are understood. To a certain extent the findings from our thematic analysis of focus group data with young men, trans/masculine, and non-binary people point towards tensions with regard to views about pregnancy and potential future parenthood. For some participants, there was a tension between endorsing the reproductive rights of other men, trans/masculine, and non-binary people, and the perception that participants had been subjected to pronatalist expectations, or that pregnancy invited a prurient focus on men, trans/masculine, and non-binary people's bodies. Additional tensions were evident in discussions about masculinity and pregnancy, with some participants struggling to see pregnancy as masculine, others endorsing normatively masculinist accounts, and others still questioning what it means to think about pregnancy as masculine. These tensions about masculinity and pregnancy were then particularly acute with regard to views within trans communities about the alleged 'cost' or appropriateness of pregnant men in terms of broader social inclusion and understanding.

In some respects, these tensions all centre upon gender norms, and specifically cisgenderist expectations. As much as men, trans/masculine, and non-binary people who are considering undertaking a pregnancy must negotiate with cisgenderist assumptions about their bodies and genders, so too are cisgender men who are considering fatherhood negotiating with the cisgenderist expectation to conform to normative gender ideals that endorse not only the assumption that assigned sex determines gender, but that gender will be 'displayed' in particular normative ways. Yet as we will explore in the remainder of this chapter, while cisgenderism would appear to impact upon all people, its impact is differentially experienced. Cisgender young men, for example, may feel pressure to adopt a normative fathering role, despite their desire to enact fatherhood in new ways. Young men, trans/masculine, and non-binary people considering gestational parenthood, by contrast, may be pressured into enacting parenting roles that are normatively associated with the sex they were assigned at birth, rather than their lived sex or gender. Men, trans/masculine, and non-binary people may be subjected to pronatalist expectations based on assumptions about their assigned sex, and may see no option other than to conform to normative masculinist understandings of parenthood. As such, despite similarities between these groups, there are marked differences that have clear implications in terms of reproductive justice.

In terms of the differential impact of cisgenderism, our thematic analysis of the focus group data would suggest the importance of inclusive sexual health education for trans people. As some of our participants suggested, making a decision about reproduction required first unpacking gender boxes so that they could ascertain the extent to which cisgenderism was shaping their views on whether or not they would consider bearing children in the future. In other interview extracts not included in this chapter, some participants spoke about 'switching off' when undertaking consultations about potential fertility preservation, a form of disengagement triggered by the view that potential future reproduction was too normatively gendered to be palatable. Inclusive sexual health education that unpacks normative gendered assumptions about reproduction, and which opens up alternate ways of thinking about future parenthood, thus holds the potential to increase the likelihood that trans people can be actively engaged with decision making about fertility, rather than simply 'switching off'.

The findings from the thematic analysis reported in this chapter also present a novel angle on the topic of sexualization, as introduced in the first chapter of this book. In the first chapter of this book we explored how trans people are alternately desexualized (i.e., in the historical expectation that trans people presented themselves as asexual to medical professionals), or hypersexualized (i.e., in the assumption that trans women specifically transition in order to be sexually desirable to men). In this chapter we explored how men, trans/masculine, and non-binary people may feel subjected to prurient focus on their bodies, a prurient focus that one participant noted constitutes a form of fetishization. This finding illustrates how reproductive and sexual justice are interconnected: that both reproductive and sexual rights centre on the right to freedom from public scrutiny of one's private decisions. For men, trans/masculine, and non-binary people, this right to privacy is particularly fraught by ongoing prurient public focus on trans people's lives and bodies.

Both the point above about the need for inclusive sexual health education, and the impact of a prurient focus on trans people's bodies, highlight how cisgenderism potentially shapes trans people's reproductive imaginaries. For some people, pregnancy may be eschewed for fear of how other people may respond. Pregnancy may be eschewed for fear of what it might say about a person's gender. Both constitute significant barriers to genuine reproductive autonomy. That, as some participants suggested, trans people who undertake pregnancies may be further marginalized within trans communities illustrates the significant costs of cisgenderism to reproductive autonomy. Challenging cisgenderism requires the types of open conversations that our participants engaged in: conversations that seek to unpack cisgenderism and its costs. Our findings would suggest that such conversations need to occur with regard to public discourse, professional practice, and also within trans communities. Specifically, in countries where trans reproductive rights are enshrined in law and public policy, conversations about cisgenderism constitute one avenue through which to pursue reproductive justice: to explore potential barriers to the enactment of reproductive rights, barriers constituted by cisgenderism.

In conclusion, in this chapter we have demonstrated how cisgenderism potentially impacts upon the reproduction autonomy of young men, trans/masculine, and non-binary people specifically, and trans people more broadly. We have highlighted how young men, trans/masculine, and non-binary people's reproductive imaginaries are shaped by three interrelated factors: (1) pronatalism, (2) cisgenderism, and (3) normative ideals about masculinity. That these three factors appear to be enforced both within and from without trans communities demonstrates their ongoing regulatory force. As such, trans reproductive justice requires a continued focus on unpacking each of these three factors, and exploring alternate ways of thinking about reproductive intentions, bodies, and the relationship between gender, gender expression, and parenthood.

References

Bartholomaeus, C., & Riggs, D. W. (2020). Intending fathers: Heterosexual men planning for a first child. *Journal of Family Studies, 26*, 77–91.

Braun, V., & Clarke, V. (2006). Using thematic analysis in psychology. *Qualitative Research in Psychology, 3*(2), 77–101.

Carpenter, E., & Niesen, R. (2021). "It's just constantly having to make a ton of decisions that other people take for granted": Pregnancy and parenting desires for queer cisgender women and non-binary individuals assigned female at birth. *Journal of GLBT Family Studies, 17*, 87–101.

Charter, R., Ussher, J. M., Perz, J., & Robinson, K. (2018). The transgender parent: Experiences and constructions of pregnancy and parenthood for transgender men in Australia. *International Journal of Transgenderism, 19*(1), 64–77.

Connell, R. W., & Messerschmidt, J. W. (2005). Hegemonic masculinity: Rethinking the concept. *Gender & Society, 19*(6), 829–859.

Corea, G. (1985). *The mother machine: Reproductive technologies from artificial insemination to artificial wombs*. New York: Harper & Row.

Edley, N., & Wetherell, M. (1999). Imagined futures: Young men's talk about fatherhood and domestic life. *British Journal of Social Psychology, 38*(2), 181–194.

Fischer, O. J. (2021). Non-binary reproduction: Stories of conception, pregnancy, and birth. *International Journal of Transgender Health, 22*, 77–88.

Hoffkling, A., Obedin-Maliver, J., & Sevelius, J. (2017). From erasure to opportunity: A qualitative study of the experiences of transgender men around pregnancy and recommendations for providers. *BMC Pregnancy and Childbirth, 17*(2), 332.

Hunter, S. C., & Riggs, D. W. (2020). *Men, caregiving and the media: The dad dilemma*. New York: Routledge.

Landau, J. (2012). Reproducing and transgressing masculinity: A rhetorical analysis of women interacting with digital photographs of Thomas Beatie. *Women's Studies in Communication, 35*(2), 178–203.

Light, A. D., Obedin-Maliver, J., Sevelius, J. M., & Kerns, J. L. (2014). Transgender men who experienced pregnancy after female-to-male gender transitioning. *Obstetrics & Gynecology, 124*(6), 1120–1127.

Marsiglio, W., Hutchinson, S., & Cohan, M. (2000). Envisioning fatherhood: A social psychological perspective on young men without kids. *Family Relations, 49*(2), 133–142.

Pascoe Leahy, P., & Bueskens, P. (Eds.). (2019). *Australian mothering: Historical and sociological perspectives*. New York: Palgrave.

Riggs, D. W. (2013). Transgender men's self-representations of bearing children post-transition. In Green, F. & Friedman, M. (Eds.), *Chasing rainbows: Exploring gender fluid parenting practices* (pp. 62–71). Toronto: Demeter Press.

Riggs, D. W. (2014). What makes a man? Thomas Beatie, embodiment, and "mundane transphobia". *Feminism & Psychology, 24*(2), 157–171.

Riggs, D. W., & Bartholomaeus, C. (2020a). "That's my job": Accounting for division of labour amongst heterosexual first time parents. *Community, Work and Family, 23*, 107–122.

Riggs, D. W., & Bartholomaeus, C. (2020b). Towards trans reproductive justice: A qualitative analysis of views on fertility preservation for Australian transgender and non-binary people. *Journal of Social Issues, 76*, 314–337.

Riggs, D. W., Pfeffer, C. A., Pearce, R., Hines, S., Ray White, F. (2021). Men, trans/masculine, and non-binary people negotiating conception: Normative resistance and inventive pragmatism. *International Journal of Transgender Health, 22*, 6–17.

Ryan, M. (2009). Beyond Thomas Beatie: Trans men and the new parenthood. In R. Epstein (Ed.), *Who's your daddy? And other writings on queer parenting* (pp. 139–150). Toronto: Sumach.

Tasker, F., & Gato, J. (2020). Gender identity and future thinking about parenthood: A qualitative analysis of focus group data With transgender and non-binary people in the United Kingdom. *Frontiers in Psychology, 11*, 865.

Thompson, R., & Lee, C. (2011). Fertile imaginations: Young men's reproductive attitudes and preferences. *Journal of Reproductive and Infant Psychology, 29*(1), 43–55.

Thompson, R., Lee, C., & Adams, J. (2013). Imagining fatherhood: Young Australian men's perspectives on fathering. *International Journal of Men's Health, 12*(2), 150–165.

Vincent, B., Erikainen, S., & Pearce, R. (Eds.). (2020). *TERF wars: Feminism and the fight for transgender futures*. London: Sage.

Wallace, J. (2010). The manly art of pregnancy. In K. Bornstein & S. Bear Bergman (Eds.), *Gender outlaws: The next generation* (pp. 188–94). San Francisco, CA: Seal Press.

10
CONCLUSION

Damien W. Riggs, Shoshana Rosenberg, Jane M. Ussher and Kerry H. Robinson

Introduction

In this book we have taken up the injunction voiced by Tuck (2009) to move beyond 'damage-centred' approaches to understanding the lives of people marginalized by social norms. Our focus on cisgenderism as one particular social norm has allowed us, in differing ways across the chapters in this book, to place responsibility for the reproductive and sexual health challenges that trans people face squarely on an ideology that seeks, either actively or passively, to deny trans people's existence. Focusing on cisgenderism as an ideology, then, is one way to resist damage-centred approaches: it doesn't deny the harmful effects of cisgenderism, but it nonetheless situates it as external to trans people, and situates it as an ideology, like any other ideology, that can be challenged

In terms of challenges to cisgenderism, in this book we have repeatedly emphasized the resistances that trans people mount to cisgenderism in both reproductive and sexual health contexts. Such resistances and the agency that informs them is also central to moving beyond a damage-centred approach. Again, focusing on the harms caused by cisgenderism is important, but equally important is focusing on how trans people speak back to, resist, and rework cisgenderism to their own ends. Rather than expecting trans people to, for example, claim damage in the face of cisgenderism in order to access healthcare services, we might instead focus on how trans people successfully access healthcare services through advocacy and through allyship with trans-inclusive providers. In other words, expecting people to emphasize harms caused as a primary mechanism for accessing care only serves to maintain a damage-centred focus.

In many of the chapters in this book, then, we have explored how trans people narrate their lives on their own terms: how trans people assert reproductive and sexual agency, including through a focus on both rights and justice. As we

DOI: 10.4324/9781003138310-10

highlighted in the first chapter of this book, while the former is important, the latter is what really gets the job done. Rights ensure that trans people are *allowed* to do certain things, but a focus on reproductive and sexual justice helps to ensure that trans people can *actually do* the things they want to do. Moreover, in the absence of rights in certain geopolitical contexts, a focus on justice helps to ensure that trans people can assert agency to navigate cisgenderist laws and healthcare systems to ensure their needs are met. Indeed, in many ways the history of trans reproductive and sexual health is a history of a focus on justice serving as a pathway, in some contexts, to legislative change. In other words, it is through a fundamental focus on the humanity of trans people that trans people and those in allyship with them have advocated for legislative and social change that helps to provide some level of protection against cisgenderism.

Taking up the points above about moving beyond a damage-centred approach to trans reproductive and sexual health, and toward a focus on trans-inclusive care that recognizes trans people's right to self-determination, in the following section we return to each of the substantive chapters of this book to map out some core principles that are likely to help ensure reproductive and sexual justice for trans people in healthcare contexts. Having outlined these core principles, we then briefly explore some areas of trans reproductive and sexual health that were not canvassed in the substantive chapters of this book, but which require concerted focus into the future.

Core principles derived from previous chapters

Chapter 2 covered the topic of pleasure in its broader conception as well as in its relation to transness. We considered the actioning of pleasure as a core aspect of resistance to the encroaching issues which affect not only our relationship with sex and sexuality, but our personal and collective lives. Our discussion explored the ways shame, the perennial counterpoint to pleasure, has been weaponized against queer and trans peoples' sexuality. As a counterpoint, this chapter offers a perspective on how these barrages of shame have been reappropriated by queer and trans peoples' as a means of self-protection and community building. This means utilizing precisely that which proponents of displeasure have used against us in our favour; relishing in what is considered shameful, seeing socially constructed borders as invitations for investigation, and ultimately reforming our relationships with our bodies, genders, and their sexual relationalities. This chapter resists the positioning of trans sexuality and pleasure as a dangerous topic or a slippery slope. Instead, we use this chapter to propose trans pleasure as a learning moment for all those who engage with it. By witnessing the processes trans peoples undergo in order to live authentically, thrive, and reimagine ourselves as people and communities under even the most dire of circumstances, readers are invited to consider their relationship to pleasure, shame, cisnormativity, and individualism.

Chapter 3 covered sexual violence experiences of trans women, from an intersectional perspective. We outlined that trans women experience sexual violence at rates significantly higher than all other groups in the community, which compounds the chronic stress experienced by trans people within a heterosexist and transphobic society. Trans women of colour face discrimination and violence based on the intersection of gender, sexuality, and racial identities. This chapter gave voice to trans women of colour living in Australia, who reported that "sexual violence is everywhere", manifested by public mockery, sexual harassment, and sexual assault, during and after gender affirmation. Heterosexual men were the primary aggressors, reflecting transmisogyny, where being trans and a women stand as multiple and intersecting risk factors for sexual violence. We demonstrated that appearing visibly different heightens the risk of violence for trans women, with the threat of sexual violence serving as gender policing. This is amplified for trans women of colour, who are simultaneously hypervisible as a trans woman and as a non-white person in a country dominated by constructions and impositions of cisgender white femininity in all areas of life. This chapter illustrates the ways in which the poor health outcomes experienced by many trans women are closely associated with exposure to sexual violence. Sexual violence is recognized to be an urgent public health priority – this chapter argues that we need to ensure that the experiences and needs of trans women are addressed in public health responses.

Chapter 4 examined experiences of sexual healthcare, as well as experiences of interactions with healthcare professionals, in relation to the mental health and wellbeing of trans and gender diverse people. We discussed the fact that trans and gender diverse people report significantly worse mental health outcomes than cis people, as a direct result of the high rates of marginalization and discrimination they experience in cis-heteronormative societies. This chapter outlined that trans and gender diverse people also have lower self-reported health compared to the general cis population and are at a high risk for both sexually transmitted infections (STIs) and blood-borne viruses (BBVs), including HIV. However, TGD people often avoid obtaining healthcare services due to their fears of being judged, or previous experiences of stigmatization, with a direct result on mental and physical health outcomes. In a survey of 699 trans and gender diverse people, we found that comfort in healthcare settings, and comfort discussing sexual health, significantly predicted self-reported mental health, suggesting mental health was better for individuals who were more comfortable discussing sexual health with HCPs. We discussed the fact that gender affirmation has positive benefits for mental health and wellbeing, producing feelings of gender euphoria. It is important that medical gender affirmation is readily available for trans and gender diverse people who choose this option. This chapter demonstrates that equitable access to sexual health services is a human rights issue for TGD people. Sexual and reproductive justice requires that TGD people should feel safe and comfortable when seeking healthcare, and should be treated with dignity and respect by clinicians.

Chapter 5 outlined the experiences of trans men who had experienced gestational pregnancy. We discussed the fact that many healthcare providers (HCPs) and the broader community position trans male pregnancy as a social and medical 'emergency' or attempt to legislate the relinquishing of trans reproductive rights. Many countries require trans people to undergo sterilization to attain legal recognition of their gender, policies described as 'passive eugenics' and HCPs may refuse to facilitate pregnancy for trans male patients. Drawing on the experiences of 25 trans men, we highlighted the ambivalent feelings around pregnancy that can be experienced, as pregnancy is associated with femininity; however, parenthood can be positively negotiated post gender affirmation. Living without testosterone during pregnancy can be difficult, as can the embodied changes during pregnancy and chest feeding. This can produce feelings of gender dysphoria for trans men. Some trans men feel isolated and socially excluded during pregnancy and after childbirth. This chapter demonstrates that education of HCPs regarding trans pregnancy is necessary to counteract the lack of knowledge in this area and to stem the discrimination that prevails.

Chapter 6 highlighted the importance of trans children's and young people's access to relevant, targeted, and co-designed information and resources about reproductive and sexual health. The sexuality education that they currently access in schools, which is framed within heteronormative cisgender discourses, does not meet the needs of trans young people, and is often anxiety provoking for them. The chapter also raised the need for greater research which includes trans children's and young people's perspectives on their reproductive futures. This will provide invaluable information about the needs of trans children and young people regarding the relevant information they require to address concerns they may have about sexuality, fertility, fertility preservation, relationships, and family formations. What this chapter shows is that these are areas of concern for many trans young people, including children. Providing safe and supported spaces where trans young people can access information about these topics and discuss them openly with knowledgeable educators and health professionals is crucial to their health and wellbeing.

Chapter 7 demonstrated the importance of understanding the cancer survivorship and cancer caring experiences of trans people, in order to develop culturally safe cancer information and care. Cancer and cancer caring may have significant and enduring negative impacts on trans cancer survivors' gender identity and expression. For others, cancer treatments or cancer caring can serve to facilitate the process of gender affirmation and increase gender euphoria. However, if HCPs operate within a cis-heteronormative framework, and do not understand the meaning of embodied change following cancer treatment for trans individuals, these positive benefits may not be realized. There is a need for HCPs to be aware of the higher risk of distress of trans cancer survivors and their carers, in particular the intersection of cancer with trans identity and embodiment, difficulties in disclosure of identity and the impact of invisibility in healthcare. HCPs have responsibility for facilitating disclosure with their patients, as many trans patients are too fearful to disclose, or are concerned that they will receive negative responses. This chapter demonstrates that specific training in offering trans-inclusive and affirmative cancer care as part of basic communication training and ongoing professional development is essential

Chapter 8 highlighted the importance of gender neutral language in the provision of reproductive healthcare. Specifically in the context of trans young people and fertility preservation counselling, using gender neutral language such as 'gametes' may help to ensure that young people actually engage with information provided. To do otherwise may be to reduce the likelihood of gaining informed consent, particularly if people disengage from information provision that they find dysphoria inducing (such as language about gametes associated with assigned sex). More broadly, and as we explored in Chapter 1, many trans people re-gender descriptions of their bodies so as to make a claim to language that reflects their gender. Rather than insisting upon using language associated with assigned sex to describe body parts, healthcare professionals aiming to implement trans-inclusive practices should check in with patients about the language they use to describe their bodies.

The topic of language was also salient in Chapter 9, highlighting clear implications for how trans people's bodies are referenced. It is common to see the assertion that, for example, 'male' and 'female' are terms referencing sex, and 'man' and 'woman' are terms referencing gender. This type of policing of language denies trans people's experiences of their bodies. For example, it is entirely appropriate for a trans man to refer to his body as male and his sex as male. He is, after all, a man. While in some healthcare contexts it may be important to ensure that information about *assigned* sex is recorded (i.e., to ensure that transmasculine people have access to pap smears or that transfeminine people have access to prostate exams), this is different to recognizing the agency of trans people to self-determine how they will be described. More broadly, in research the tendency to refer to people's bodies according to assigned sex has negative implications. Referring to trans men, for example, as having 'female genitals' again denies the reality of such men's lives and experiences, thus constituting a form of cisgenderism. Given how fraught healthcare experiences can be for many people, especially with regard to misgendering, a move away from resorting to language associated with assigned sex is likely to at the very least help healthcare professionals to remain focused on a person's gender/ sex as they determine it.

Additional areas of focus for the future

Abortion remains very much a live issue for people across the globe, with some countries removing laws that prevent access to abortion, while other countries have further implemented laws that restrict or prevent access to abortion services. Given the fraught status of abortion services, it is no surprise that trans-inclusive abortion services remain even more fraught. Limited services, or the perception or reality of cisgenderist service provision, leads some trans people to engage in abortion attempts without clinical supervision. Moseson et al. (2021), for example, found that of the 1694 trans people they surveyed, 40 (19% of those who had ever been pregnant) reported self-managed abortions, including through the use of herbs, physical trauma, or substance use. Given the potential for considerable negative outcomes, self-management of abortions for trans people is highly concerning.

Even for trans people who do access abortion services, their experiences are not great. Fix et al. (2020), for example, found that abortion services that use language focused on cisgender women can be a significant barrier for trans people seeking to access services. Some participants noted that limited knowledge among providers about trans-inclusive practice also translated into less than optimal experiences. By contrast, Lowik (2018) provides a comprehensive resource for abortion service providers, outlining key aspects of trans-inclusive care. Key to such services is the use of trans-inclusive language. This starts with services using language such as 'pregnant people', or 'people who require an abortion', rather than referring solely to women. Following through on the use of inclusive language also requires visual representations that are inclusive of trans people. This can include on the service website (so not only images of women), in pamphlets (again, which should use inclusive language as per above), and in promotional materials. All such documents should clearly state that trans people are welcome in services. Also in order to facilitate inclusion, thought should be given to the clinical space. Given most waiting rooms for abortion services will primarily serve cisgender women, transmasculine people may feel uncomfortable in this space. When scheduling an appointment, services should consider offering trans people the use of a private or screened-off waiting area. Also, in terms of the clinic space, services should ensure that gender neutral or men's toilets are available.

In a similar way, the provision of information about menstruation is too often focused on cisgender women, thus failing to meet the needs of many trans people. For trans people who menstruate, the provision of inclusive information about menstrual suppression can be vital for helping to alleviate dysphoria (Lowik, 2021). Yet many trans people who menstruate face challenges in accessing trans-inclusive services, such as with regard to having a mirena installed, or receiving medication that can stop menstruation. Trans people in Lowik's study reported that when they sought to access surgeries that would remove their reproductive organs, they were told that they should want to preserve their reproductive capacity, but also were questioned under the guise that surgeries aimed at ceasing menstruation were viewed by some healthcare providers as a backdoor way of accessing gender affirming surgeries. If people who menstruate find it difficult to access services, then it is understandable that trans people who do not menstruate may find it especially difficult to share their experiences. As Lowik found, for example, some trans women report psychological and physical experiences akin to menstrual cycles, yet this is rarely spoken about by healthcare professionals.

On a related topic, research (e.g., Gezer et al., 2021) suggests that trans people might be more likely to experience polycystic ovarian syndrome (PCOS), yet treatments for PCOS (often involving hormones) may compound dysphoria experienced by some trans people (Bell, 2018). For other trans people, while the pain of PCOS may be acutely distressing, aspects of PCOS (such as body hair growth) may be welcomed, though for some people it may be an additional cause of distress (Bell, 2018). Anecdotally, and similar to the findings of Lowik (2021), some trans people may struggle to access surgery to treat PCOS, as it may be viewed as a backdoor way of accessing gender-affirming care that isn't otherwise covered by social healthcare in countries where this is available. More attention is thus needed to how trans people experience PCOS, and healthcare services must actively engage with the specific needs of trans people living with PCOS.

Another area which requires further attention is trans peoples' experiences and potential challenges with regard to contraception. Current research remains unclear regarding the impact of HRT on trans peoples' ability to either conceive or avoid conception (Mancini et al., 2021). While many trans peoples believe that HRT is in and of itself a form of contraception, trans men and other transmasculine people have been shown to be capable of becoming pregnant even well into their medical transition (Abern & Maguire, 2018; Light et al., 2018). Even less is known about trans women and transfeminine peoples' capacity for conceiving following hormone therapy, as most studies are focused on people capable of giving birth, though the few studies in this area suggest that sperm production persists even in people who have been on oestrogen-based hormone treatments long term (Jiang et al., 2019).

With regards to contraception methods such as condoms and PrEP, the uptake of these methods remains lower than average within many trans communities (Callander et al., 2019; Nieto et al., 2021; Reisner et al., 2021), largely due to structural and cultural barriers regarding the ways these contraception methods are accessed and promoted. This has repercussions in terms of STI rates, which are significantly higher for trans peoples compared to their cisgender counterparts (Andrzejewski et al., 2021; Nematollahi et al., 2021). As with other issues discussed above, a foundational barrier to proper STI prevention methods is structural cisgenderism and its impact on sexual health education, testing, and contraceptive use uptake (Rosenberg et al., 2021). The path forward in terms of promoting safer sex practices within trans communities therefore requires a multi-pronged approach, countering the ways transphobia, stigma, miseducation, and socioeconomic factors converge to form this cluster of issues.

Another aspect of safe sexual practice we were unable to explore in this book is chemsex. Although some studies cover sexualized drug use in the context of trans communities (e.g. (Jalil et al., 2022)), most research in the area tends to either focus on cis gay men's experiences or otherwise aggregates trans and cis peoples' experiences under the banner of "LGBT communities" (Hibbert et al., 2021; Jaspal, 2021). It is important to consider chemsex in all its complexity, including its role in subcultural and interpersonal expressions of resistance to heterosexual normativity (Mowlabocus, 2021) as well as its negative ramifications, such as its correlation with HIV transmission (Tan et al., 2021) and its potential to facilitate non-consensual sexual encounters (Drückler et al., 2021). Chemsex as a phenomenon is therefore necessary to be explored in the context of trans peoples, particularly considering its connection with issues that significantly affect trans communities. However, this investigation needs to be done carefully, with mindfulness of the stigma that is often inherent in discussions of sexualized drug use. In particular, while chemsex can be problematic (Maxwell, 2021), it can also facilitate inter- and intrapersonal sexual experiences which cannot be achieved otherwise. It would do more harm than good to research trans peoples' experiences of chemsex without this balanced perspective, particularly when considering the many positive aspects of chemical use that trans people experience throughout their lives e.g., HRT.

With all these considerations around sexual health in mind, it is important to note that more emphasis needs to be placed in future literature around the intersections of transness, sexuality, and disability. Disabled trans peoples face multi-layered barriers when it comes to community access writ large (Ramasamy, Rillotta, & Alexander, 2021), as well as experiencing a higher likelihood of victimization as a result of their intersecting experiences (Messinger, Guadalupe-Diaz, & Kurdyla, 2021). Disabled peoples are also excluded from comprehensive and trans-inclusive sexual health education, both in terms of the accessibility of these materials and their inclusion of disability-specific topics (Tarasoff, 2021; Ubisi, 2021). As both transness and disability have the potential to radically transform any areas of life they intersect with (Hettinga et al., 2021), it is vital to consider the nexus of disability, transness, and sexuality. As shown in this book, trans sexuality can be a space for significant reimaginings and recomprehensions of normative sexual narratives. Similarly, the meeting space between disability and sexuality is fertile ground for new understandings of sexuality (Godin-Jacques, 2021). We hope to provide more room for exploring the triangulation of these factors in future writings.

Another area not addressed substantively in this book is the topic of sex work. It is commonly stated that due to challenges in gaining other forms of employment, and compounded by the fetishization and marginalization of trans people's bodies, many trans people engage in sex work. Certainly, it is true to say that for many trans people, and perhaps particularly for trans women of colour, sex work is often framed as a 'survival sex', a form of work that is not simply precarious, but for many people is connected to serious harms including violence, HIV transmission, and for some people death (Nadal, Davidoff, & Fujii-Doe, 2014; Sausa, Keatley, & Operario, 2007). While we would not for a moment want to discount or minimize a focus on such harms, resisting a damage-centred account of sex work by and for trans people requires an additional area of focus on agency and empowerment. Australian research with Indigenous transmasculine and transfeminine people, for example, highlights how sex work enables some people to resist racism, and to assert agency in the face of social marginalization (Sullivan, 2018; Sullivan & Day, 2019). This suggests that studies of trans reproductive and sexual justice must continue to strive to pair the effects of social marginalization – including here in terms of precarity and the ways in which it may force people into survival sex – with the agency that trans people enact in the face of such marginalization, including in terms of engaging in sex work.

Finally, we would note that more work is needed to explore tensions between reproductive and sexual justice for trans people, and the marketization of services. Specifically, we would note that while it is vital that trans people have access to reproductive services, this is different to trans people being targeted as consumers of reproductive services. It is one thing for services to ensure that they are trans inclusive, and another thing for trans people to be seen as a market to be targeted. Referred to as 'extractivism' (Wichterich, 2019), the focus on any given population group as a potential 'market' does very little to actually ensure the needs of the given population are met, and instead focuses on finding ways to increase market share and thus produce profit. Moreover, an extractivist logic may mean that people are pushed into services (or service 'add-ons' in the context of reproductive care) that do not meet their needs, or which upsell their needs over and beyond other possible low-tech options. Certainly, within a reproductive justice approach trans people should have the right and capacity to make decisions about services. But this should be led by the needs and desires of trans people, not by the desires of the market.

Conclusions

In this book we have argued for a trans-specific reproductive and sexual justice approach. Across genders, age cohorts, life experiences, and cultural groups we have argued that trans people experience unique reproductive and sexual needs, shaped broadly by cisgenderism, but specifically by individual social locations. Nonetheless, more work needs to be done to further map out a diversity of experiences within trans communities when it comes to reproductive and sexual justice, especially given that both are founded in movements led by women of colour (National Latina Institute for Reproductive Health, 2013; SisterSong, 2003; Smith, 2005). As cárdenas (2016) notes, for trans women of colour in particular, reproductive and sexual justice encompasses not simply the right to make decisions about one's life and to have the capacity to enact one's decisions, but also the right simply to be alive to make decisions in the first place. The same is true across a diversity of experiences including but not limited to ability, religion, cultural context, and age.

Vital to ensuring a continued focus on trans reproductive and sexual justice are the clinical contexts through which trans-inclusive care is provided. Given the historical moment at which this book was written, specifically referencing here the awaited release of the World Professional Association for Transgender Health's eighth edition of their Standards of Care (SOC), it was not possible to speak to how the latest iteration of the Standards will address trans reproductive and sexual justice. Certainly we know that previous iterations (alongside iterations of both the Diagnostic and Statistical Manual (DSM) and the International Classification of Diseases) have been problematic in terms of speaking to the rights of trans people, let alone to the topic of justice (Riggs et al., 2019). Nonetheless, we remain optimistic that into the future a concerted focus on reproductive and sexual justice will come to take centre stage.

In response to ongoing transnormative and pathologizing approaches to clinical care for trans people, trans people have sought to develop affirming approaches to clinical research and practice that challenge the broader disciplinary regulation of their lives. Key to affirming clinical approaches has been the recent development of the informed consent model of care, developed and implemented in partnership with trans people (e.g., Cundill & Wiggins, 2017). Rather than centring clinician diagnosis and authorization for treatment, this model of care emphasizes that trans people are more than capable of authorizing their own treatment in collaboration with clinicians (Schulz, 2018). Such an approach challenges traditional models of care as outlined in the DSM and SOC, which in many instances in their application continue to gatekeep access to care. Furthermore, an informed consent model recognizes that, in many cases, trans people know more about their needs than many clinicians, given the dearth of training and specialization in the field of transgender health.

Lacking, however, is the application of informed consent models in the context of reproductive and sexual health. Primarily such models have been utilized when trans people seek to access hormone therapies. An informed consent model may be equally useful when it comes to thinking through how access to reproductive and sexual healthcare services is facilitated. This would involve centring the knowledges that trans people have about their reproductive and sexual health needs, knowledges that are community-led and shaped by the agency of trans people. Situating these knowledges alongside those of trans-affirming clinicians (and trans clinicians themselves) can provide or create pathways to reproductive and sexual healthcare that are trans led, and which challenge traditional gatekeeping and pathologizing approaches.

In conclusion, this book speaks to both strengths and challenges, agency and marginalization, and potentials and pitfalls in the context of trans reproductive and sexual health. Across the chapters we have sought to encourage an expansive focus on what constitutes reproductive and sexual health for trans people, as much as we have acknowledged above other areas that require concerted focus into the future. The futures that we imagine when it comes to trans reproductive and sexual justice are only constrained by our willingness to challenge cisgenderism, and our capacity to examine which voices dominate in the study of trans people's lives, and to work towards the creation and celebration of spaces where trans people's voices dominate. Ultimately, while as Ansara and Hegarty (2013) have noted, the trans/cis binary is itself a problem that limits our understanding of all people's lives, as we have highlighted across this book, a focus on the unique reproductive and sexual health needs of trans people is nonetheless very much needed, so as to counter cisgenderism and foster spaces for gender euphoria.

References

Abern, L., & Maguire, K. (2018). Contraception knowledge in transgender individuals: Are we doing enough?. *Obstetrics & Gynecology, 131*, 65S.

Andrzejewski, J., Dunville, R., Johns, M. M., Michaels, S., & Reisner, S. L. (2021). Medical gender affirmation and HIV and sexually transmitted disease prevention in transgender youth: Results from the survey of today's adolescent relationships and transitions, 2018. *LGBT Health, 8*(3), 181–189.

Ansara, Y. G., & Hegarty, P. (2013). Misgendering in English language contexts: Applying non-cisgenderist methods to feminist research. *International Journal of Multiple Research Approaches, 7*(2), 160–177.

Bell, J. (2018). What it's like to have PCOS when you're trans. Retrieved from https://helloclue.com/articles/cycle-a-z/what's-it-like-to-have-pcos-when-you're-trans

Callander, D., Wiggins, J., Rosenberg, S., Cornelisse, V., Duck-Chong, E., Holt, M., & Cook, T. (2019). *The 2018 Australian trans and gender diverse sexual health survey: Report of findings*. Sydney, NSW: The Kirby Institute, UNSW Sydney.

Cárdenas, M. (2016). Pregnancy: Reproductive futures in trans of color feminism. *Transgender Studies Quarterly, 3*(1–2), 48–57.

Cundill, P., & Wiggins, J. (2017). *Protocols for the initiation of hormone therapy for trans and gender diverse patients.* Melbourne: Equinox Gender Diverse Clinic. Retrieved from https://equinox.org.au/resources/

Drückler, S., Speulman, J., van Rooijen, M., & Vries, H. J. C. D. (2021). Sexual consent and chemsex: A quantitative study on sexualised drug use and non-consensual sex among men who have sex with men in Amsterdam, the Netherlands. *Sexually Transmitted Infections, 97*(4), 268–275.

Fix, L., Durden, M., Obedin-Maliver, J., Moseson, H., Hastings, J., Stoeffler, A., & Baum, S. E. (2020). Stakeholder perceptions and experiences regarding access to contraception and abortion for transgender, non-binary, and gender-expansive individuals assigned female at birth in the US. *Archives of Sexual Behavior, 49*(7), 2683–2702.

Gezer, E., Piro, B., Cantürk, Z., Çetinarslan, B., Sözen, M., Selek, A., ... & Seal, L. J. (2021). The comparison of gender dysphoria, body image satisfaction and quality of life between treatment-naive transgender males with and without polycystic ovary syndrome. *Transgender Health.* http://doi.org/10.1089/trgh.2021.0061

Godin-Jacques, C. C. (2021). *Who's at the table? The homogenization of crip queers in decision-making and policy-making processes.* M.A., Queen's University (Canada). Retrieved from www.proquest.com/docview/2616346389/abstract/51E6909BE2654DCFPQ/1

Hettinga, L., Buikema, R., Quinan, C., Thiele, K., University Utrecht, Faculteit Geesteswetenschappen, & Gender Studies. (2021). *Appearing differently: Disability and transgender embodiment in contemporary Euro-American visual cultures.* Utrecht University. Retrieved from https://dspace.library.uu.nl/handle/1874/415752

Hibbert, M. P., Hillis, A., Brett, C. E., Porcellato, L. A., & Hope, V. D. (2021). A narrative systematic review of sexualised drug use and sexual health outcomes among LGBT people. *International Journal of Drug Policy.* https://doi.org/10.1016/j.drugpo.2021.103187

Jalil, E. M., Torres, T. S., de A Pereira, C. C., Farias, A., Brito, J. D. U., Lacerda, M., da Silva, D. A. R., Wallys, N., Ribeiro, G., Gomes, J., Odara, T., Santiago, L., Nouveau, S., Benedetti, M., Pimenta, C., Hoagland, B., Grinsztejn, B., & Veloso, V. G. (2022). High rates of sexualized drug use or chemsex among Brazilian transgender women and young sexual and gender minorities. *International Journal of Environmental Research and Public Health, 19*(3), 1704.

Jaspal, R. (2021). Chemsex, identity processes and coping among gay and bisexual men. *Drugs and Alcohol Today, 21*(4), 345–355.

Jiang, D. D., Swenson, E., Mason, M., Turner, K. R., Dugi, D. D., Hedges, J. C., & Hecht, S. L. (2019). Effects of estrogen on spermatogenesis in transgender women. *Urology, 132,* 117–122.

Light, A., Wang, L.-F., Zeymo, A., & Gomez-Lobo, V. (2018). Family planning and contraception use in transgender men. *Contraception, 98*(4), 266–269.

Lowik, A. (2018). *Trans-inclusive abortion services: A manual for operationalizing trans-inclusive policies and practices in an abortion setting.* Retrieved from www.ajlowik.com/publications#/transinclusive-abortion

Lowik, A. (2021). "Just because I don't bleed, doesn't mean I don't go through it": Expanding knowledge on trans and non-binary menstruators. *International Journal of Transgender Health, 22*(1–2), 113–125.

Mancini, I., Alvisi, S., Gava, G., Seracchioli, R., & Meriggiola, M. C. (2021). Contraception across transgender. *International Journal of Impotence Research, 33*(7), 710–719.

Maxwell, S. (2021). *Pre-exposure prophylaxis use among men who have sex with men who have engaged in chemsex.* Doctoral thesis, University College London (UCL), pp. 1–190. Retrieved from https://discovery.ucl.ac.uk/id/eprint/10134742/

Messinger, A. M., Guadalupe-Diaz, X. L., & Kurdyla, V. (2021). Transgender polyvictimization in the U.S. Transgender Survey. *Journal of Interpersonal Violence*. https://doi.org/10.1177/08862605211039250

Moseson, H., Fix, L., Gerdts, C., Ragosta, S., Hastings, J., Stoeffler, A., … Obedin-Maliver, J. (2021). Abortion attempts without clinical supervision among transgender, nonbinary and gender-expansive people in the United States. *BMJ Sexual & Reproductive Health*.

Mowlabocus, S. (2021). Fucking with homonormativity: The ambiguous politics of chemsex. *Sexualities*. https://doi.org/10.1177/1363460721999267

Nadal, K. L., Davidoff, K. C., & Fujii-Doe, W. (2014). Transgender women and the sex work industry: Roots in systemic, institutional, and interpersonal discrimination. *Journal of Trauma & Dissociation*, *15*(2), 169–183.

National Latina Institute for Reproductive Health. (2013). *At the margins of care: The need for inclusive health care for transgender and gender non-conconforming Latin@s*. New York: National Latina Institute for Reproductive Health.

Nematollahi, A., Gharibzadeh, S., Damghanian, M., Gholamzadeh, S., & Farnam, F. (2021). Sexual behaviors and vulnerability to sexually transmitted infections in transgender women in Iran. *BMC Women's Health*, *22*, 1–8.

Nieto, O., Fehrenbacher, A. E., Cabral, A., Landrian, A., & Brooks, R. A. (2021). Barriers and motivators to pre-exposure prophylaxis uptake among Black and Latina transgender women in Los Angeles: Perspectives of current PrEP users. *AIDS Care*, *33*(2), 244–252.

Ramasamy, V. (Resh), Rillotta, F., & Alexander, J. (2021). Experiences of adults with intellectual disabilities who identify as lesbian, gay, bisexual, or transgender within mainstream community: A systematic review of qualitative studies. *JBI Evidence Synthesis*, *19*(1), 59–154.

Reisner, S. L., Moore, C. S., Asquith, A., Pardee, D. J., & Mayer, K. H. (2021). The pre-exposure prophylaxis cascade in at-risk transgender men who have sex with men in the United States. *LGBT Health*, *8*(2), 116–124.

Riggs, D.W., Pearce, R., Pfeffer, C., Hines, S., White, F., & Ruspini, E. (2019). Transnormativity in the psy disciplines: Constructing pathology in the *Diagnostic and statistical manual of mental disorders* and *standards of care*. *American Psychologist*, *74*, 912–924.

Rosenberg, S., Callander, D., Holt, M., Duck-Chong, L., Pony, M., Cornelisse, V., Baradaran, A., Duncan, D. T., & Cook, T. (2021). Cisgenderism and transphobia in sexual health care and associations with testing for HIV and other sexually transmitted infections: Findings from the Australian Trans & Gender Diverse Sexual Health Survey. *PLOS ONE*, *16*(7), e0253589.

Sausa, L. A., Keatley, J., & Operario, D. (2007). Perceived risks and benefits of sex work among transgender women of color in San Francisco. *Archives of Sexual Behavior*, *36*(6), 768–777.

Schulz, S. L. (2018). The informed consent model of transgender care: An alternative to the diagnosis of gender dysphoria. *Journal of Humanistic Psychology*, *58*, 72–92.

SisterSong. (2003). *SisterSong reproductive health and sexual rights national conference program book*. Atlanta, GA: SisterSong Women of Color Reproductive Health Collective.

Smith, A. (2005). Beyond pro-choice versus pro-life: Women of color and reproductive justice. *NWSA Journal*, *17*(1), 119–140.

Sullivan, C. T. (2018). Majesty in the city: Experiences of an Aboriginal transgender sex worker in Sydney, Australia. *Gender, Place & Culture*, *25*(12), 1681–1702.

Sullivan, C. T., & Day, M. (2019). Indigenous transmasculine Australians and sex work. *Emotion, Space and Society*, *32*, 100591.

Tan, R. K. J., Phua, K., Tan, A., Gan, D. C. J., Ho, L. P. P., Ong, E. J., & See, M. Y. (2021). Exploring the role of trauma in underpinning sexualised drug use ('chemsex') among gay, bisexual and other men who have sex with men in Singapore. *International Journal of Drug Policy*. https://doi.org/10.1016/j.drugpo.2021.103333

Tarasoff, L. A. (2021). A call for comprehensive, disability- and LGBTQ-inclusive sexual and reproductive health education. *Journal of Adolescent Health*, *69*(2), 185–186.

Tuck, E. (2009). Suspending damage: A letter to communities. *Harvard Educational Review*, *79*(3), 409–428.

Ubisi, L. (2021). Addressing LGBT+ issues in comprehensive sexuality education for learners with visual impairment: Guidance from disability professionals. *Sex Education*, *21*(3), 347–361.

Wichterich, C. (2019). *Care extractivism and the reconfiguration of social reproduction in post-Fordist economies*. International Center for Development and Decent Work Working Papers, Paper No. 25.

INDEX

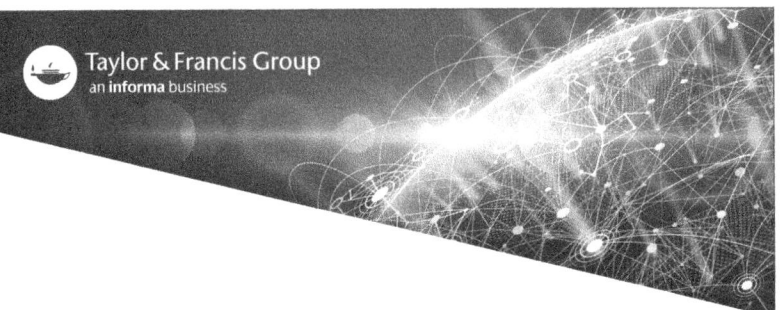

Taylor & Francis Group
an **informa** business

Taylor & Francis eBooks

www.taylorfrancis.com

A single destination for eBooks from Taylor & Francis
with increased functionality and an improved user
experience to meet the needs of our customers.

90,000+ eBooks of award-winning academic content in
Humanities, Social Science, Science, Technology, Engineering,
and Medical written by a global network of editors and authors.

TAYLOR & FRANCIS EBOOKS OFFERS:

A streamlined
experience for
our library
customers

A single point
of discovery
for all of our
eBook content

Improved
search and
discovery of
content at both
book and
chapter level

REQUEST A FREE TRIAL
support@taylorfrancis.com

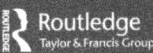 Routledge
Taylor & Francis Group

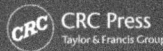 CRC Press
Taylor & Francis Group